Complete Calisthenics

Complete Calisthenics
The Ultimate Guide to
Bodyweight Exercise

Ashley Kalym

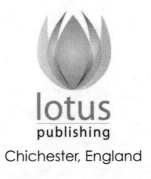

lotus
publishing

Chichester, England

First published in 2014 through CreateSpace (9781495425271).
This revised edition published in 2014 by
Lotus Publishing
Apple Tree Cottage, Inlands Road, Nutbourne, Chichester, PO18 8RJ

Photographs Chris Frosin
Text Design Mary-Anne Trant
Cover Design Mike Seymour
Printed and Bound in the UK by Short Run Press Limited

British Library Cataloguing-in-Publication Data
A CIP record for this book is available from the British Library
ISBN 978 1 905367 54 2

Disclaimer
The material contained in this book is for informational purposes only. The author and anyone else affiliated with the creation or distribution of this book may not be held liable for damages of any kind whatsoever allegedly caused or resulting from any such claimed reliance. Before beginning this or any workout routine, it is recommended that you consult with a qualified physician for authorisation and clearance. It is always recommended to consult with a physician before beginning any new exercise or nutritional program. If you have any problems with your health, you should seek clearance from a qualified medical professional. The information contained herein is not intended to, and never should, substitute for the necessity of seeking the advice of a qualified medical professional. If at any time you feel pain or discomfort, stop immediately. Parts of this book contain advanced exercises that should not be attempted until you are ready.

All efforts have been made to ensure that this manual is free from error or problems. Although we have worked hard, we do not take responsibility for loss or action to any individual as a result of the material presented here.

Contents

Part IV: The Exercises

Part V: Training Programs

Preface

The journey I have taken to the point of writing this book has been long and varied. I started my bodyweight exercise journey when I was very young: with the persuasion of my parents, I was enrolled into junior rugby and began to get a taste of physical training. Being too young to work with weights, we trained with push-ups, pull-ups, sit-ups, lunges, and a lot of running around to get our bodies into shape. This was not just due to the fact that we were too young; the club I played for really didn't have the money or the facilities to let us train with weights, so for a long time I knew of no other method of training. After several years of this, I was old enough to begin training using weights and weighted exercise. I then did the traditional thing of bicep curling, chest exercises, doing lat pull downs instead of pull-ups, and using the leg extension machine instead of actually squatting. I gained some muscle during this period, but one component that was missing from my physical development was real strength. Even after using weights for a number of years, I wasn't actually strong, and the lesson that really brought that home was to come in a few years' time.

After leaving university I had a few jobs, and then decided that the time was right to try and enter the Royal Marine Commandos. It was a massively daunting task, and as soon as I read through the paperwork and the brochure I was somewhat surprised to find training in the military was all about using bodyweight to build a strong, fatigue-resistant physique. So, whilst in training I found myself doing the same exercises that I had done when I had been much younger, namely push-ups, pull-ups, running, and other simple bodyweight movements. I entered the military in early 2009 and found my physical preparation with bodyweight exercise had been well worthwhile. After about eight months I decided that the military life and lots of time away from home wasn't for me, so I decided to come back to civilian life. I had learnt so much whilst I was in training, mostly about myself and where my limits lay, and I was also hugely impressed with how fit and strong I had become by performing simple bodyweight exercises. It was in one of those moments that I decided I wanted to see how strong I could become using bodyweight training, so I started to research anything I could get my hands on about that form of exercise.

After a number of weeks I eventually stumbled across a website of short tutorials on some of the more basic gymnastic elements, like the back lever, muscle-up, and so on. I gave them a go, and utterly failed. Undeterred, I decided that the best place to try and learn how to increase my strength was a gymnastic class. So, I booked myself onto one, went along, and was again absolutely humbled. Here were children, not more than ten or eleven years old, performing bodyweight strength movements that I could not even fathom. Even the simplest core exercise that they were working with (the half lever, or L sit) absolutely crushed my core, and I remember going away with all of my preconceived notions of strength and bodyweight training in pieces. From that moment, I decided to pursue calisthenic training as far as it could possibly take me. Other commitments also meant that I did not have the spare forty hours a week needed to train to be a gymnast. However, I did have a desire to become strong, really strong, and I knew that the secret lay in progressive bodyweight exercise.

The next few years were a huge learning experience, and they were also some of the most exciting training times that I have ever been through. Almost every week I was learning something new, coming across a groundbreaking piece of information, an innovative technique or method of building strength, and my limits were pushed again and again. Slowly, I began to create my own methods of progression, and taking what was good from other programs and developing a solid regimen of my own.

Then, I began to look for a book that compiled all the knowledge I had gained, showing how to progress from a complete beginner to someone who had almost inhuman strength. I looked and looked but couldn't find anything. There were some books on bodyweight training, but these were mostly simple affairs, only concerned with teaching the reader how to perform the most rudimentary exercises, e.g. the push-up or the sit-up. Others were a little more comprehensive but missed out lower body training completely. Therefore, I set out to write a book to help anyone, male or female, beginner or advanced, to build strength, athleticism, power, and an incredible physique using just their bodyweight. *Complete Calisthenics* is that book.

Every method to achieve awesome bodyweight strength is presented, with an explanation of calisthenics, its benefits and drawbacks, to the equipment you will need, and even a section on the correct nutrition. In the exercise section you will learn how to perform movements like the humble push-up, all the way through to triceps dips, handstands, muscle-ups, front levers, one-arm pull-ups, human flags, and single-leg squats. Each exercise is demonstrated with a number of clear, instructive photographs, enabling you to see exactly what your body should be doing at each stage. To conclude, there is an extensive description of various training programs, suitable for total beginners as well as those of you who have been training for years. Wherever you are now on your journey, this book will give you the tools and motivation you need to take your physical training to the next level. In short, *Complete Calisthenics* is the ultimate guide on how to develop the ultimate bodyweight strength.

Acknowledgements

There are many people I wish to thank and many people who have helped me over the last few years, not all of them knowingly. First I wish to thank my friend Phil Taylor for encouraging me to pursue this avenue of training. I wish to thank Mitch Edwards, who shared his knowledge and expertise from the moment I set foot into the world of gymnastic conditioning. On the web I wish to thank Jim Bathhurst from Beastskills.com, whose tutorials and articles have taught me so much. I would like to thank Coach Christopher Sommer of Gymnasticbodies.com, who provides advice and encouragement and asks for little in return, and lastly to the myriad of YouTube users who have provided insight, inspiration, and much, much more.

I would also like to thank Chris Frosin, who has been an invaluable part of my journey to becoming a writer, and whose patience and expertise made this book possible. His website can be found at the following link: **www.chrisfrosin.co.uk**

For cover design and visual inspiration, I would like to thank Mike Seymour, again whose patience and zest for design has encouraged me more than once. His blog and portfolio can be found at the following link: **www.behance.com/sey**

I would like to thank Sam and the awesome guys at Rigs Fitness in Birmingham for the use of their gym. After asking what seemed like countless people, Sam stepped up and could not have been more helpful or accommodating. They have an amazing world-class set-up and can be found on the web at the following link: **www. rigsfitness.co.uk**

The most important thank you is to you, the reader, without whom I would not be able to continue to do something that I love for a living, and without whom the world of calisthenics would not be as bright. Thank you for purchasing this book. It was a pleasure to write, gave me many late nights, but it was definitely worth it!

If you would like to get in touch, or have any questions or comments, then please send me an email at the following address: **completecalisthenicsuk@gmail.com**

I endeavour to reply to every email in person, and look forward to hearing from you.

Train hard!

Ashley Kalym

Introduction

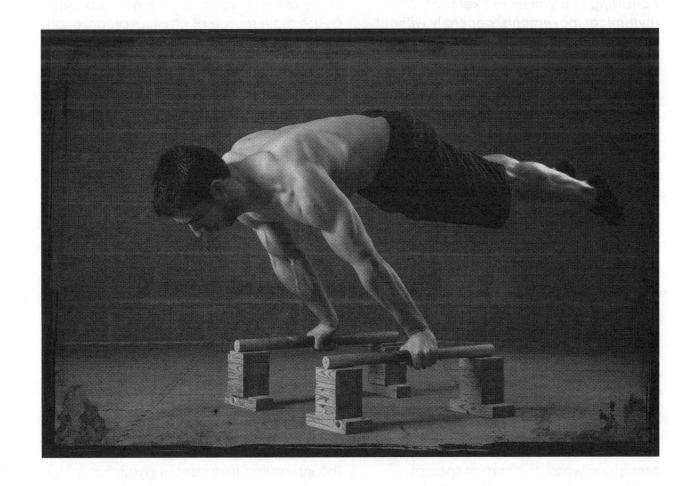

1 What Is Calisthenics?

Firstly, it is worth taking a look at exactly what calisthenics is, and what it isn't, so that we know why certain exercises are included or excluded.

The word 'calisthenics' comes from the ancient Greek 'kallos', which means beauty, and 'sthenos', which means strength. It can be thought of as the art of using your own bodyweight and qualities of inertia as a means to develop your physique. Wikipedia, defines calisthenics as follows:

Calisthenics is a form of physical training consisting of a variety of exercises, often rhythmical movements, generally without using equipment or apparatus. They are intended to increase body strength and flexibility with movements such as bending, jumping, swinging, twisting or kicking, using only one's body weight for resistance. They are usually conducted in concert with stretches. Calisthenics when performed vigorously and with variety can benefit both muscular and cardiovascular fitness, in addition to improving psychomotor skills such as balance, agility and coordination.

Groups such as sports teams and military units often perform leader-directed group calisthenics as a form of synchronized physical training to increase group cohesion and discipline. Calisthenics are also popular as a component of physical education in primary and secondary schools around the world.

The history of calisthenics stretches back to the dawn of human evolution. In the prehistoric world, the human species walked, ran, jumped, lunged, climbed, pushed, and pulled as part of their everyday activity and the struggle to survive. Modern weights and machines that are found in commercial gyms are light years away from the kind of activity that we humans have been engaged in for millennia, and this is why, in my opinion at least, calisthenics is the most natural and comfortable type of exercise and movement for us to perform. Our cousins, the great apes, make use of this to develop huge strength in the upper body, as is evident when watching chimpanzees climb trees and swing from branch to branch with ease.

In the ancient world, calisthenics was used as the main source of physical preparation for the military, as it was easy to organise, easy to learn, and had the biggest transfer to the actual skills and movements that soldiers would need. There is also something spiritual about being in tune with one's own body, and being able to move it through space with no limits or barriers. Technology also limited what was possible, as barbells, specific weights, and weighted movements were not understood. Then, as now, physical strength was revered and admired, as the legends of Milo, Atlas, and Hercules attest. These famous and mythical figures were known for one key attribute, and that was their strength and ability to exert force using their muscles.

Today's pinnacle of calisthenic-type movement is without doubt the elite gymnast. If there is another athlete that is pound for pound stronger, more agile, more powerful, more flexible, or more mobile, then I have yet to hear of them. The interesting thing about gymnasts is that their strength can almost be thought of as a by-product, as they normally train exclusively for their event or discipline, and not for the ability to be strong. Even though this is the case, most gymnastic training takes place behind closed doors, and many train upwards of thirty to forty hours per week, which for many people is simply not possible with the lives that they lead. In addition, much of gymnastic training is traditionally done with the aim of eventual progress and perfecting specific disciplines that a particular gymnast will compete in. For the person who just wants to be able to perform one-arm pull-ups, or a front lever, the majority of gymnastic training might be wasted on them, and not everyone can commit or has the discipline to train as a gymnast does.

In recent years calisthenics has really seen a huge leap forward, in terms of its popularity and the movements being performed. Anyone reading this who is familiar with YouTube will no doubt have seen many amazing videos where ordinary people display acts of inhuman strength and muscular control, using equipment no more advanced than a pull-up bar. This is the essence of calisthenics: using the body to perform feats of strength that are rarely seen in other training disciplines.

Another fascinating and admirable characteristic of modern calisthenics is that most of the people who are involved in this type of training do not pay for a gym membership, do not have access to expensive equipment, and do not have people telling them exactly what to do. In principle, they train in parks and basements, on pull-up bars and dip bars that they may have constructed themselves, yet they have more strength than the majority of muscle heads that populate many commercial gyms. As a result of this, it is no surprise to see that calisthenics also has a large place in parkour or free running culture. These men and women perform feats of strength

and daring as they run, jump, climb, push, and pull themselves over, under, and through street obstacles using grace and athleticism. Nearly all of these people are very well versed in calisthenics and body weight strength movements as well, which makes this book ideal for those who are beginning free running or parkour. In the last few years, specialist workout competitions have become popular, where very strong men and women compete against each other on a street workout course. Some of the movements displayed here would not be out of place on an international gymnastic arena, such is the level of strength and athleticism shown.

Finally, calisthenics is also used as a strength building tool for other sports, as it serves to build a foundation that is not really available anywhere else. Even other types of athlete, like the Olympic Weightlifter, perform rudimentary calisthenic movements to build a base level of strength before diverging and performing sport-specific examples. The name that most comes to mind is that of the 77kg World and Olympic champion Weightlifter Lu Xiaojun. This is a man who can snatch 176kg and clean and jerk 204kg, but for whom calisthenic and bodyweight exercise is a regular staple in his training routine. He can be seen in many videos and pictures performing handstand push-ups, human flags, weighted dips, and other movements that would not look out of place in a street workout.

Advantages of Calisthenics

Now that we have seen exactly what calisthenics is, it is time to look at the advantages of this method of training.

Everyone can do calisthenics

Firstly, everybody is somewhat accustomed to performing bodyweight exercise, as they have been moving their own bodyweight through space since the day they were born. In addition, the resistance is tailor-made for each individual as their own bodyweight is used as the resistance. I have often found that many people easily take to training with calisthenics when compared to handling dumbbells and barbells for the first time. This is good because it increases confidence and motivation. I cannot tell you how many times I have informed a client that we will be working with push-ups, only for them to tell me that they cannot do them. Five minutes later, after I teach them exactly how to perform a simplified variation, their face lights up as they realise that they are perfectly capable of performing calisthenics, even if it is at a beginner level.

A safe form of exercise

Secondly, compared to many other forms of exercise, it is not easy to injure yourself performing calisthenics for the simple reason that to increase resistance requires the leverage or range of motion to be manipulated. This is not true with dumbbell and barbell exercises however, where even complete novices can add extremely large amounts of weight, resulting in a greatly increased risk of injury. In addition, a lot of the more difficult exercises in calisthenics simply cannot be performed unless they are worked up to over a period of months

and years before they can be attempted and trained regularly. Compare this to weighted movements, where even a beginner can put 100kg or 200lbs on a bar and attempt to squat with it.

Exercise difficulty is scalable

Thirdly, the difficulty of each calisthenic exercise can be made more challenging by altering the leverage that can be brought to bear on the movement. At first this concept can be hard to understand. To increase the resistance in nearly all other forms of exercise, more weight is simply added to the bar or a heavier weight is picked up and moved. But as we are using calisthenics we cannot simply add more bodyweight. To increase the resistance we have to make it more difficult for the muscles to apply force. To illustrate this point, think about holding a heavy dumbbell or similar object in your hand, with the weight hanging by your side. The weight in question lies directly under your shoulder musculature, making it very easy to hold the position. Now imagine slowly raising the weight out to the side, keeping your elbow locked. This position would become increasingly difficult to hold, until the exercise would become most difficult to hold with the arm horizontal. At this point the ability of the shoulder muscles to exert force on the weight is reduced, which results in more strength being needed to hold the position. This makes the muscle stronger over time, even though the actual weight lifted has not changed. This concept of manipulating leverage of an exercise is used extensively in this book, especially for the more demanding movements. As you progress through the book you will notice that exercises like the front lever, back lever, pseudo planche push-up, and many others, all rely on this method of manipulating leverage to increase the difficulty of the exercise.

Transferable strength

Fourthly, the strength built using calisthenics is transferable to a wide range of sports and athletic pursuits. There are many theories that attempt to explain this, and all may be equally valid. My own personal opinion is that nearly all calisthenic movements, and especially the more advanced ones, teach the body how to work as a complete unit. If we take the planche as an example, this exercise requires all of the muscles in the body to act as one, with complete tension required in order for the movement to be performed. This is especially useful because weighted exercises and barbell and dumbbell movements are not suitable for some people, especially the young and undertrained. Using calisthenics enables anyone to develop a solid foundation of strength from which to progress.

Builds unique types of strength

Finally, calisthenics makes ample use of isometric exercises. Isometric exercises are those where the muscles are under tension without becoming shorter or longer. Pushing against a locked door or solid wall would be a real-world example of an isometric contraction. This is unlike concentric contractions, where the muscles become shorter under tension, or eccentric contractions, where the muscles become longer under tension. Isometric exercises are different to normal exercises because repetitions are not counted, and instead the exercise is held for a set amount of time. There is no real way to replicate isometric calisthenic exercises with weights, and the type of strength that can be built with these locked, static positions is unique. This is because for all of the isometric exercises, the body has to contract all of the muscles as hard as possible at the same time. This means more muscle is involved in the exercise, which means more strength can be built. An example is the half lever, which is shown below.

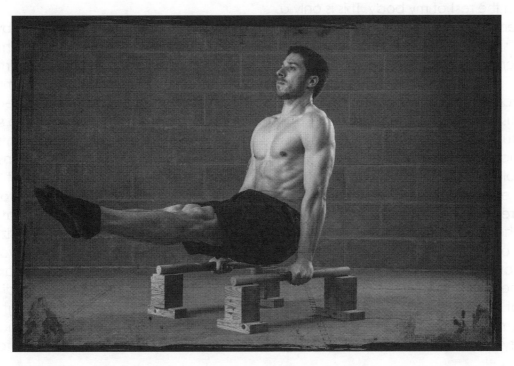

Disadvantages of Calisthenics

Even though there are many benefits to performing calisthenics, there are a few drawbacks as well, and it is worth considering these before we progress.

• Since no weights are used it can be difficult to build massive strength in the lower body using just your own bodyweight as the resistance. The lower body is home to the biggest and most powerful muscle groups in the body, such as the quadriceps and glutes. This means that they need to contract against a lot of resistance to elicit any strength gains. Unfortunately there are not a great number of calisthenic exercises that we can use to provide enough resistance to build huge lower body strength. Bodyweight squats, single-leg squats, lunges, and hamstring curls are some of the exercises we will look at later in the book, and although these build huge amounts of strength, I personally found that when starting to train with Olympic Weightlifting and back and front squats, my legs were far behind the rest of my body. This is only a concern of course if lower body strength or the specific ability to squat large loads is important to you.

• The second disadvantage is that because of the way the lower body is constructed, it is hard to design exercises that incorporate decreased leverage principles. The upper body is home to many exercises that rely on this concept to increase strength gains, such as the planche, the front and back lever, and many others. There is no way around this fact, which is why on nearly every calisthenic's video, the person either will not look like he trains legs, or will not perform any lower body exercises. This is a pity in my opinion, because training the lower body can help enormously in muscle building and strength gains in the rest of the body.

• The third drawback is that as weight cannot be added to increase resistance, except in the case of weighted pull-ups, etc. then we have to rely on the method of decreasing the amount of leverage to make the movement more difficult. Whilst this is an extremely effective way of making an exercise more challenging, it is not the same as increasing the load on a barbell by a few kilograms or pounds every few weeks. For example, if we were doing the bench press, we could quite accurately keep track of exactly how much weight we were lifting and how much it was increasing by each week or month. For calisthenics we cannot do this. We can of course keep a record of the number of repetitions, how much our range of motion changed by, and how long we held certain positions, but calisthenic training is a lot less accurate in terms of recording progress.

• The fourth drawback is disputed by some people but nevertheless remains a popular opinion, which is that performing calisthenics cannot build lots of muscle. I do not think this is true, simply because of the size of some people I have seen performing calisthenic movements. A quick look on YouTube will demonstrate that there are some seriously built individuals doing nothing apart from bodyweight exercise. It is true that there is probably a limit to the muscle size that calisthenics can give you, but if you want bodybuilder size then it would make sense for you to just do bodybuilding. If you want serious, inhuman strength, as well as good size and amazing muscle tone, then calisthenics is the way forward.

Unique Aspects of Calisthenics

As calisthenics is a unique form of training and exercise, it has its own unique benefits and traits, and I would like to spend some time now taking a look at them. These aspects are down to the way in which calisthenic exercises use the muscles of the body, as well as the equipment, or lack of it, that is used. This means that calisthenics can be used to develop types of strength and athleticism that cannot be developed elsewhere or using other methods.

Hand Strength

The first unique aspect of calisthenics is that the hands are involved in almost every single movement that we will look at. Pushing, pulling, and core exercises all use the hands to a large degree and, because calisthenics puts an emphasis on complete control and all over body strength, aids like straps and hooks are not used at all. This is in contrast to bodybuilding and other weighted forms of exercise, where straps are used to help people hang onto pull-up bars, and hooks are used to help hold the barbell when dead lifting. No doubt you will have seen this being done in gyms by nearly everybody that is trying to become strong. For the bodybuilder, using hooks and straps is part and parcel of the sport; they are trying to target certain muscles and they do not want the hands and forearms to tire before the main muscle group they are working on becomes fatigued. However, we as calisthenic practitioners want the hands and the forearms, and by extension the grip, to be as strong as physically possible. This makes perfect sense if you give it a moment's thought. You could have the strongest back in the world, but if your hands and forearms are not strong enough to transfer that strength and make use of it,

it is pointless. I am such a believer in hand strength that I have written an entire book, called *Grip*, on the subject.

In calisthenics you use your hands for many purposes: holding yourself on the floor and manipulating your bodyweight, gripping a pull-up bar and hanging from apparatus, and moving from one position to another using pure strength and not momentum. All of these rely on hand and finger strength and without them, you will simply not be able to perform some of the more advanced calisthenic movements. There are of course specific hand and finger strength exercises that can be used to directly target the muscles used for gripping, but much of the strength needed can and will be gained by simply performing the standard exercises that I have laid out in Part IV.

Core

The core is a part of the body that has seen its fair share of fad exercises and gadgets over the years, and I think we can all safely say that the majority of these are an absolute waste of time, energy and money. Contrary to popular belief, or what the media may tell you, a strong core will not be built by doing thousands of sit-ups or crunches. Nor will performing crunches and sit-ups burn any fat from your mid section. The core musculature is no different from any other muscle fibre in terms of what it needs to become stronger. To become stronger, a muscle needs to contract against a resistance, and in order for that strength to grow, the resistance needs to increase over time. **It is not the amount of repetitions that needs to increase, it is the resistance.** This means that no matter how many sit-ups you do, your body will not become stronger if you fail to increase the resistance.

In traditional exercise the core is seen as simply a body part to be aesthetically improved. The abs are worked on, diet is adhered to religiously and all people want a six-pack. However, in calisthenics the core plays a vital role and is not just relegated to the back seat. Many exercises that can be called calisthenic require the core to keep the midline of the body absolutely stable. If we take an exercise such as the front lever, we can see that even though it is hugely reliant upon upper body pulling strength, the core also has to keep the whole body straight and hold up the weight of the legs. This means that a core built using calisthenic exercises will be among the strongest you are ever likely to encounter.

As we have to increase the resistance in order to increase strength this means that we have to dispense with a lot of the more traditional core exercises. This is not to say that this book does not contain easier core movements, it does, but just those alone cannot be relied upon to build the core strength we need if we are to progress to a decent level.

The more advanced core exercises, many of which you may not have seen before, such as the half lever, are very common in gymnastic circles. They build such huge core strength, which once perfected, make other core exercises seem like child's play. Be in no doubt that once you can perform some of the more advanced movements, you will be able to rightly claim to having one of the strongest cores around.

Scapula

Of all the regions of the body that are involved in calisthenic movements, especially the advanced ones, muscular support of the scapula is perhaps the most important. While many eager practitioners focus on big chests and large backs, the real key to upper body strength is the ability to stabilise and control the scapula.

Through its attachment to the clavicle, the scapula provides a bony anchor for the arm to the rib cage. It is also a bony anchor for many of the key muscles (for example: serratus anterior, all three divisions of the trapezius, and rhomboids) that are largely responsible for providing stability for the upper extremity.

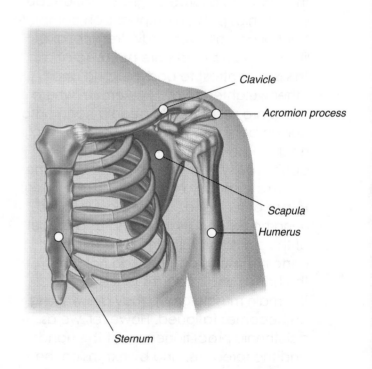

Clavicle

Acromion process

Scapula

Humerus

Sternum

If the muscles that stabilise the scapula have been well-developed through proper conditioning, force generated through the upper extremities can be transferred into optimal movement with much greater efficiency.

There are six primary directions of scapular movement: elevation, depression, upward and downward rotation, and protraction and retraction. Elevation occurs when you shrug your shoulders up, or move your shoulders to your ears. Depression occurs when you let your shoulders sink down towards the ground. Upward rotation occurs as you reach the arm overhead and the glenoid fossa faces up towards the sky while downward rotation occurs as you bring your arm back from the overhead position. Retraction occurs when you adduct and pull your shoulders back while lifting your chest up and protraction occurs as you reach your arms forwards and pull shoulder blades away from the spine.

The scapula is also an important muscular attachment point for the muscles of the glenohumeral (ball and socket) joint including the deltoid and rotator cuff. The glenohumeral joint has been analogously described as a golf ball sitting on a golf tee. The rotator cuff muscles are therefore particularly important in maintaining glenohumeral joint stability through a wide range of activities.

These four muscles arise from the scapula and connect to the head of the humerus forming a cuff at the shoulder joint. Along with the long head of the biceps brachii, they are the muscles primarily responsible for stabilising the head of the humerus upon the relatively small and shallow glenoid fossa of the scapula.

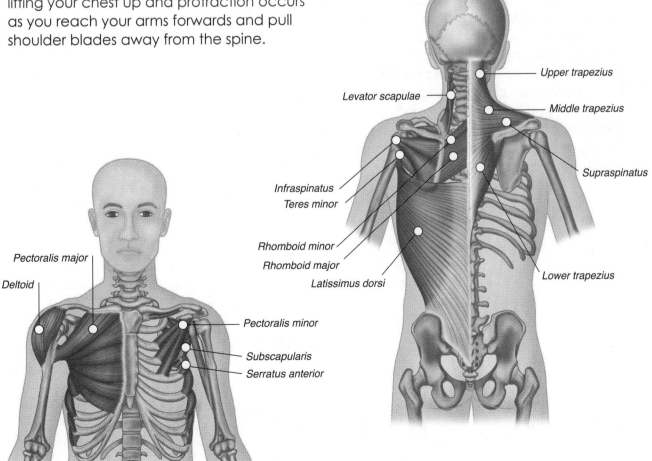

Pectoralis major
Deltoid
Pectoralis minor
Subscapularis
Serratus anterior

Levator scapulae
Upper trapezius
Middle trapezius
Supraspinatus
Infraspinatus
Teres minor
Rhomboid minor
Rhomboid major
Latissimus dorsi
Lower trapezius

In addition to stabilising the glenohumeral joint and controlling humeral head translation, the rotator cuff muscles also play an important role in shoulder rotation. The *infraspinatus* and *teres minor* both externally rotate the shoulder and tend to translate the humeral head forwards on the glenoid fossa. This action is counteracted by the *subscapularis*, which internally rotates and posteriorly translates the humeral head upon the glenoid fossa. However, working synergistically, these muscles are important for maintaining an optimal axis of rotation of the glenohumeral joint during shoulder movement.

Shoulder abduction is initiated by the *supraspinatus*. This is accomplished by contraction of the supraspinatus, which translates the humeral head inferiorly to enable the humeral head to rotate under the acromion process. Because the deltoid is a larger and stronger muscle, it often becomes dominant and drives the humeral head up pinching the supraspinatus tendon under the acromion process. This is a common cause of supraspinatus or 'rotator cuff impingement' and generally causes pain when lifting the arms overhead or performing common calisthenic patterns.

This is a key point for your success in performing many of the most difficult calisthenic movements: you must be able to maintain optimal control both of the scapula and glenohumeral joint so that the larger muscle groups, such as the pectorals, latissimus dorsi, and deltoids, can perform the actual movement patterns. This concept holds especially true for pull-ups, planches, front levers, one-arm chin-ups, and many other exercises that require extreme strength. In the mobility section of the book I will detail several exercises that are essential for shoulder health that should be performed by everyone, regardless of your starting level of strength.

Text supplied with grateful thanks, by Evan Osar, author of *Corrective Exercise Solutions to Common Hip and Shoulder Dysfunction* (2013).

Straight-Arm Strength

Calisthenics, and by extension much of gymnastics, places heavy emphasis on a phenomenon known as straight-arm strength. Even if you are not familiar with this concept you will have no doubt seen it being used. Gymnasts use it when performing movements on the still rings, for example the iron cross or crucifix, or when displaying their planche skills.

Straight-arm strength is exactly what it sounds like: strength exerted with a locked elbow. This puts enormous strain on the arm and its connective tissues, including the biceps and the biceps tendon, and also the hands and the wrists. Movements like the planche, which we will examine in detail later on in the book, make use of straight-arm strength without which it would be difficult or impossible to perform. This feat is also the reason why many gymnasts and calisthenic practitioners have very large biceps, even though they do no traditional biceps curl exercises of any kind. The tension on the elongated muscle makes it increase in size and strength dramatically, and also makes many of the more advanced calisthenic exercises possible.

Another excellent side effect of using a straight arm to pull with is that it makes the back extremely strong. If the arm is kept straight then the muscles in the back have to work extremely hard to exert any force on the bar. This obviously increases strength in a way that cannot be replicated with any other method. This is also the reason why calisthenic and gymnastic practitioners have incredible back musculature. In this book there are a number of exercises that rely on straight-arm strength. The planche, front lever, back lever, and human flag are just some of the movements that will expose you to this novel and unique aspect of calisthenics.

Training the Nervous System

Another very unique aspect of calisthenics, which is only really felt when performing very intense workouts, is that of the nervous system being trained. This is best felt rather than described, but is simply the body being taxed and stressed so much that you feel as though more than just your muscles have been worked. This facet of calisthenics is experienced most when working with the movements that involve lots of muscle groups simultaneously, or that require lots of muscular tension to be held for extended periods. Examples of this are the planche, the front, back, and half levers, and very difficult movements like the one-arm pull-up. You will find that you cannot simply keep performing repetitions of these exercises indefinitely, as the body becomes fatigued and drained after only a short while. This is normal, and is simply a sign that the exercise is doing its job.

This is also seen in strongman training, powerlifting and weightlifting. Imagine going for a one rep max deadlift. An exercise such as this requires so much force to be produced that you simply cannot keep performing it over and over again. You may be able to continue for a couple of repetitions but after that your body will become very fatigued. This is exactly the same thing that happens with the high-level calisthenic movements, but simply using bodyweight exercises.

Equipment

The beauty of using a method of exercise like calisthenics is that there is almost no equipment that is required for you to perform the workouts. You can often find all that you need to have an extremely effective calisthenic workout in any playground or play park: as long as it is deemed suitable for you to train, you can find pull-up bars, dip bars, vertical bars, monkey bars, and many other pieces of equipment. In some countries there are even specialist workout areas with many different types of bar set-ups, including varying heights and thicknesses. These are rare however.

This is not to say that you can use just any equipment to perform movements and exercises. Other books I have seen dealing with bodyweight exercise recommend using household objects extensively in your workouts. This is a very bad idea for a number of reasons, primarily because the vast majority of household objects are not designed for doing pull-ups, dips, or other exercises. So if they fail or break whilst you are using them, you may become injured.

Calisthenics also has the added bonus that it should be very cheap for you to acquire the equipment and apparatus you need. Most often the material that the equipment is made from is cheap, readily available, and is not complicated to build. This is in stark contrast to vibration plates, treadmills, cross trainers, rowing machines, weight plates and Olympic bars, etc., which can be extremely expensive to buy and maintain. You will notice that pull-up and dip bars do not require maintenance!

In the next few pages we will look at the different types of equipment that can be used in calisthenic training, where they can be found, and how important each piece is to your success.

Location

When starting your calisthenic training, you need to decide where to train. This is a big decision, as it is most important that you enjoy your training, and if you do not find a place that is suitable, then it is much more likely that you will give up. There are numerous locations that can be suitable, and I will run through a few suggestions here.

- Firstly, commercial gyms and health clubs can be excellent for calisthenic training and hopefully nearly everybody reading this book will live relatively close to one of these facilities. The benefits are that they normally have plenty of equipment, they are indoors so the weather will not affect your training schedule, and the prices are competitive. The downsides are that you will be paying for many facilities (like swimming pools, etc.) that you will perhaps not use. Also, the type of equipment they have will not be completely calisthenics-friendly. CrossFit gyms are very good for calisthenic training. Whatever your opinion on CrossFit, and I have many, it cannot be denied that they have some very good facilities with equipment that is pretty much perfect for those interested in doing calisthenics.

- Secondly, playgrounds and play parks are another viable option for those wishing to train using calisthenics but who do not want to join a gym, or spend any money on equipment. Most playgrounds these days have various pull-up bars, dip bars, monkey bars, poles, ropes, etc., and can be much better to use than a commercial gym. The downsides are that nearly all playgrounds and parks are outside, so if you intend on using somewhere like this for your training, you will have to contend with the weather. The other is safety. Playgrounds are designed primarily for children, and there could be issues with adults working out in close proximity to children. In this instance, it would be best to check with the local authority, and see if it would be permissible for you to train there. Alternatively, you could just wait until the children have gone home.

- Thirdly, use an area that has been specifically set-up as a bodyweight and calisthenic workout area. If you live in the United States, Eastern Europe or Russia, then these are becoming more and more common, especially within the cities, where they can normally be found next to, or joined onto, basketball courts. These are less common in the UK, but are becoming steadily more accessible, due to initiatives to get young people more active. These types of workout areas normally have a multitude of pull-up bars, dip bars, parallettes, etc., of various heights and bar thicknesses. The other excellent benefit of areas like this is that there will be other people that want to train as you do, and having training partners or being part of a group is one of the fastest ways of progressing.

- Finally, the last place that you can train is in your own home. This will require purchasing or making some equipment yourself, as it is unlikely that your home will have a ready-made calisthenic gym. This does not mean that you need to spend a fortune however, as most of the equipment needed for calisthenic training is very cheap and readily available.

Now we will look at some of the pieces of apparatus that are used for calisthenic and bodyweight training, where you can find them, and alternatives to the bought items.

Pull-Up Bar

Even though equipment is not really needed for calisthenics, it is very difficult, perhaps impossible, to perform any of the pulling exercises without something to pull on. The best piece of equipment for this is a pull-up bar. Not only can a pull-up bar be used for all of the pulling exercises, but it can also be utilised for most of the core exercises, and even some of the pushing exercises. This makes it perhaps the most cost-effective piece of exercise equipment ever devised. All gyms should have pull-up bars, and if they don't, either don't join or change gyms. If you are lucky, then they will have a bar that is not too close to the ceiling; this will allow you to progress onto muscle-ups in time. If on the other hand you are not a member of a gym, and have no intention of ever joining one, then there are a number of options open to you.

Firstly, you can buy a pull-up bar. If you go down this route then it will probably be one of the best decisions you can make on your physical training journey. Pull-up bars come in various types, from those that bolt to walls, to those that fit into doorframes, and even stand-alone units. You should be able to find one that suits your budget and living situation fairly easily. For example, I use a PowerBar* at home that I have been using dutifully for a few years now. It has never let me down, was very cheap, and seems to fit a wide variety of doorframes.

Please note that I am not endorsed or sponsored by the company that makes this particular product, I have just had a very good experience with it.

If you cannot afford a pull-up bar, or have nowhere to install one, then there are alternatives: anything that you can grab that is above your head would work. This could include the underneath of stairs in a basement or cellar, a balcony, or even a tree branch. As long as whatever you choose can support your weight safely, I see no reason why it cannot be used to perform pulling exercises on.

Dip Bars

Dip bars are another common piece of equipment found in not only commercial gyms but also in play parks and outside training areas. As the name suggests they are normally used for triceps dips, but can also be used for other types of exercises, including front and back levers, muscle-ups, handstand and planche work.

The dip bars that are found in commercial gyms are often attached to a bigger piece of equipment, like pull-up bars and leg raise stations, so sometimes these are not that suitable for a pure calisthenic workout, but can still be used effectively. In play parks the dip bars are often much longer, which means that two to three people can train simultaneously, or you can travel along them, turn around, perform handstands, planches, etc., and get a really good workout. As with pull-up bars, dip bars can come in a lot of variations, with different bar thicknesses, widths, and heights. It is rare to find stand-alone units that you can buy, but if you look on the Internet you may find some.

As I have the space in my home, I have built a set of dip bars in my back garden, and if you have the space and the spare time, I strongly encourage you to do this as well (as long as the people you may share a house with allow it of course). Building your own means that you can customise the width, height and thickness of the bars for your own body shape and type: if you are interested in doing this, a quick search on Google should bring up lots of tutorials.

Parallettes

Parallettes are similar in some ways to dip bars, in that they consist of two bars that are a set distance apart, and are facing the same way. The difference is that parallettes are normally portable and are much lower to the ground. If you have ever seen push-up bars, then parallettes are simply a larger version. Parallettes are designed for pushing exercises, such as push-ups, handstands, planche work, etc. The beauty is that as they are separate units, you can widen and narrow the grip to suit your particular body type. Also, because they are so small and portable, they can be taken almost anywhere. This is perfect if you are either away from home regularly through travel or business, or simply do not have much room in your home to build a training area.

Parallettes come in various different types but there are a few factors that you should look out for when buying them:

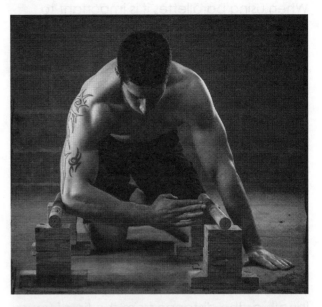

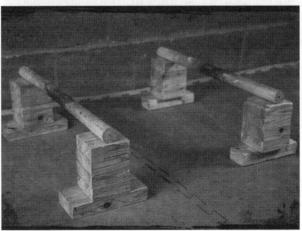

• They need to be sturdy. This is for the obvious reason that you do not want the apparatus you are using to fail, otherwise you will possibly injure either yourself or others.

• They need to have a bar thickness that is comfortable for you to hold onto. It is no good using parallettes that have a diameter of a few inches, and although that would do wonders for your grip strength, it will make handstands, planches and other exercises much more difficult to control. There are a number of places on the Internet where you can buy parallettes, so it is best to have a look around and see what you can find.

• Make your own, as I have done. This is very simple and can save you money. There are many instructional videos and

tutorials on the Internet that will show you how to make workout equipment, including parallettes. Doing a quick search should yield a good number of results, but the basic structure can be seen with my own parallettes.

As you can see, I took a single piece of thick dowel, about 1¼ inches in diameter and cut it in half. Then I stacked up small squares of wood until I had four towers, each about 10 to 12 inches high. These were then screwed together and the ends of the dowel fixed to the four towers. They obviously look very homemade, but I have had these for about five years now, and they have not failed me once.

When using parallettes it is important to make sure that they are positioned the correct width apart. This will be unique for every person; however, the simplest method is to position them shoulder width apart. This means that when you practice planches, handstands, half levers, etc., your hands will be positioned directly underneath your shoulders. This will make it much easier to support yourself, as your arms will act like vertical columns supporting the rest of your bodyweight. To find your shoulder width, you can either look at yourself in a mirror, or find a training partner to help you. If in doubt, then your shoulder width is normally the same length as the distance from the tip of your fingers to your elbow. Simply position your parallettes according to this measurement and you will be good to go.

Clothing

The type of clothing you wear is not really that important, but there are a few factors to bear in mind. Firstly, whatever you choose to wear to workout and train in should allow your body complete freedom of movement, with no restrictions at the joints. One of the ways in which strength is built in calisthenics is by using the full range of motion in every exercise so if this is restricted by the clothes that you are wearing, you will be off to a bad start. My apparel of choice is normally loose fitting shorts and a t-shirt or vest, or if I am training somewhere that allows me to go shirtless, then I will train with no shirt on.

Training with no shirt has numerous benefits, such as more freedom to move, less resistance to joint movement, and also it allows the body to regulate its temperature properly. Training with no shirt also allows you to observe your movements more closely, and to actually see what the body is doing at all times. This is invaluable because if you have a training partner, they will be able to give you feedback on any incorrect or correct movements, especially when it comes to learning and feeling the body position for exercises like the back lever, etc. Also, do not think that you need to spend a lot of money on workout clothes. Soon, you will be performing muscle-ups and other movements where the material of your clothes will come into contact with the bars and other surfaces, and this is one of the quickest ways to ruin a special t-shirt. In addition, contrary to what the big sports brands may tell you, their clothing will not turn you into a calisthenic king overnight, so do yourself a service and save some money.

Chalk

Many of the exercises in this book, especially those involving heavy use of the hands and upper body, require a very strong and secure grip. For example, the false grip, which is a technique used for muscle-ups on the pull-up bar, relies on the hands not moving from a set position, otherwise the movement will not be able to be completed successfully. To that end, it is very important to make sure your grip will not slip due to sweat from either the hands or a slippery surface on the piece of equipment. That is where chalk is important: it basically dries out the hands and creates a more abrasive and stickier surface for the grip. There are two main types of chalk:

1. The first is the traditional powdered chalk that you may have seen being used by gymnasts, weightlifters, and climbers. This normally comes in large square blocks, which are then broken down and placed in a container of some kind. The

downsides to this are many, including excess chalk on the floor and on the apparatus, chalk dust in the air which can be breathed in or make its way into the eyes, and the job of reapplying the chalk after a short period of time.

2. The second type is liquid chalk, which normally comes in a small bottle. Liquid chalk is the same compound as normal powdered chalk, except that a liquid is added that evaporates off the skin once it is applied. This leaves a thin layer of chalk over the surface of the palm of the hand, which makes the grip on pull-up bars and parallettes much stronger. Liquid chalk also does not have to be reapplied quite as often as powdered chalk, does not get into the air, lungs or eyes, and can also be applied onto the wrists and other parts of the anatomy that powdered chalk cannot.

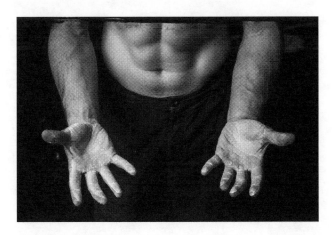

Foam Roller

Although a foam roller is not vital, it can come in handy for mobility drills and maintenance of muscle and tissue. A foam roller is used for *self myofascial* release, or more simply, *foam rolling*. Foam rolling is the act of putting pressure on a muscle or muscle group, and rolling over it using the body's own weight as the force. This can help to align muscle fibres, release the fascia from the muscle, and generally get rid of any sore parts, scar tissue, and knots in the muscle fibre.

Foam rollers can be bought from a number of sources, and most good commercial gyms should have some available. They normally come in various densities, with the softer rollers more suitable for beginners, and the harder ones more suitable for those who have already been foam rolling for some time. If you do not want to buy a foam roller solely for your training, then you can use many household objects to achieve much the same result, e.g. tennis balls, cardboard tubes, and plumbing pipes, etc.

Training Partner

The last piece of optional equipment is a training partner. Depending on your social circle and the type of people who are your friends, you will either have people lining up to train alongside you, or those who make every excuse under the sun not to exercise. If you can find someone who can take the part of a regular training partner, then you will be in luck. A training partner can really make the difference, especially in terms of pushing you to break through plateaus and to hit new highs. Often, you will find that training alongside someone else will help to promote a healthy dose of rivalry and competition, which is only ever good for progress and improvement. They will also be able to watch you exercise and tell you where you are going wrong and when you are doing things right.

Nutrition, Rest and Recovery

Now that you have an understanding of calisthenics and the type of strength that it will give you, it is time to look at a very important part of all physical training, which is nutrition, rest, and recovery. Many people make the mistake of training very hard, but then don't eat properly, rest or sleep enough, and then subsequently fail to recover and become stronger. This next part of the book aims to provide all the information you will need relating to a suitable diet, the correct amount of rest time, and the right amount and type of sleep.

If you are serious about building real strength and power, then you will need to ensure that you eat the correct amount of nutrients and are properly hydrated. (If you are interested in reading more about nutrition, please refer to the resources list on page 334; there is simply not enough space in this book to go into great detail.) Below are some basic guidelines and information.

Diet becomes even more important if you also want to reduce your body fat and get ripped. There is so much money to be made from diets, with seemingly a new one being devised daily. This means the vast majority of diets and nutritional plans out there are garbage. Many nutritionists and dieticians complicate matters far too much, in the hope that you will become reliant on their advice and expertise indefinitely. In my experience, complications only cause problems, whereas keeping it simple means any plan will be easier to follow and more successful.

Read any fitness magazine and you will see many different rules and regulations for eating a good diet. Some will say to control calories, some will advise not eating carbohydrates for the first week, and some will have traffic light systems for different foods. In my opinion all of these diets and methods of eating are more trouble than they are worth. Building serious calisthenic strength requires lots of actual training, and we do not want to waste time trying to follow an extremely complex way of eating. In this next section, I have listed a number of rules relating to diet and nutrition that are easy to follow and should make perfect sense.

Drink More Water

The vast majority of people do not drink enough water, which means that dehydration is a big problem in society. This becomes even worse when you bring training into the mix. Water is used for every process the body carries out, from the transport of nutrients around the body to the essential functions of the brain. Most places have readily available drinking water, so there is really no excuse to be dehydrated. A good tip is to take a water bottle around with you wherever you go, and take small sips often. This will ensure that you always stay hydrated wherever you may be, or whatever you might be doing.

It is no exaggeration to say that dehydration can affect performance in a very major way, especially if you are trying to become stronger, more powerful, and just simply put more effort into your workouts. If you really struggle to meet any of the other requirements in this section, then try as hard as you can to meet this one. You will also find that your skin becomes clearer, you will become less tired, and you will be able to concentrate for longer periods of time.

To evaluate how much you should be drinking, simply multiply your weight in kg by 0.033. For example, I weigh 75kg, so 75kg x 0.033 = 2.475 litres. So, I should aim to drink 2.5 litres of water a day. If you live in a hot climate or if you have trained hard, then just drink more to compensate.

Note: to work out your weight into kilos from pounds, simply divide your weight in pounds by 2.2. For example, 165lbs divided by 2.2 = 75kg.

Eat Natural Food

Natural food is that which has been minimally processed, and either walks, swims, flies, or grows. Meat, fish, poultry, eggs, nuts, fruit and vegetables are all types of natural food. This rule is very straightforward. The more natural food you eat the better, as it will contain more and better quality nutrients, and will be more suited to your body's digestive system. It is up to you whether you eat organic food or not. There is plenty of evidence to show that organic food is no better for you than non-organic food, but this makes no sense to me. I do not eat organic food exclusively, but you may want to think about this type of diet if you are concerned about pesticides and herbicides contaminating your food.

In terms of what food to eat, a mix of nutrients is best. This means meat, fish, eggs, and dairy for your protein, lots of fruits and vegetables for your carbohydrates, and your fat from meat, olive oil, nuts and seeds. Contrary to popular belief, eating an all-natural diet is not more expensive than eating junk food, and even if it was, that is still not a reason to eat junk food. It can also be thought of as the single ingredient diet. If you only eat natural food then everything you eat should consist of a single ingredient. In this regard it is the simplest diet to follow that has ever been devised. When selecting food simply hold it in your hand and ask yourself whether it has a single ingredient or not. If it does, then eat it, if it doesn't, then don't eat it. Very simple!

Eat Big To Get Big

Many of you reading this will want to put on muscle mass, either for aesthetic reasons or to make the strength exercises more manageable. To put on muscle you must simply take in more calories than you expend, but these must be good quality calories. This has often been rendered as "eat big to get big". If you are training for strength then you will undoubtedly feel the need to eat more, so do not feel guilty for doing so. Strength training is extremely taxing on the body, and food and nutrients will need to be consumed in bulk so that your body will have the materials to repair itself. We have been accustomed to hearing about daily calorie intakes for adults, and, in my opinion, these have skewed the view of nearly everyone about what constitutes a good diet. If you are training for strength then you will need to eat much more than doctors and other health professionals recommend. As an extreme example, read any interview with some of the strongest men on the planet right now: men like Brian Shaw, Benedikt Magnusson, and others, and you will often hear them say that they eat close to 10,000 calories per day. This is because when training for strength you have to eat, and you have to eat a lot.

One drawback to eating lots of food, even if it is very good quality natural food, is that there is a chance that you will put on body fat. This is unavoidable to a certain extent, which is why bodybuilders will go through a bulking and dieting phase, where in the first stage they will eat and put on muscle, and then reduce their calories and body fat. Do not worry too much about this, as once you have reached a stage where you have put on the muscle mass you want, you can reduce the amount of food you eat and drop body fat.

Increase Your Protein Intake

Out of all of the macronutrients (the others being carbohydrates and fats), protein is perhaps the most important one when training for strength. This is because protein is the nutrient that is responsible for the growth and maintenance of muscle. Eating enough food that contains protein will help you to keep the muscle that you already have, which is important for obvious reasons. Protein can be found in meat like beef, pork, and lamb, all types of fish, eggs, milk, cheese and other dairy products, and legumes, nuts, and seeds. If you eat a fairly varied diet you should have no trouble absorbing enough protein into your body, especially if you are not a vegetarian.

It is also worth understanding which types of protein are the best, as the higher quality the protein, the better your results will be. All of the research points to the fact that animal protein is the best for you, regardless of what vegetarians might think. This is not a dig at vegetarians, but simply stating a scientific fact. Animal protein is known to have a complete amino acid profile, which is good for a number of reasons, mainly that your body will be able to repair any damage done to it and not be missing any vital nutrients to do so.

How the meat that you eat is fed has a drastic effect on the quality of the food. For example, there is a huge difference between grass fed and corn fed beef. Cows have evolved to eat grass; that's what their ancestors ate, and that is what their digestive system is designed for, so when they are fed grain they have side effects, just as many people who eat gluten have side effects. The grass fed beef has much better amino acid profiles, and is much healthier for you, so if you can, try and eat grass fed beef, poultry and other meat as often as possible.

If you are a vegetarian then you can still build muscle and strength, as the example of most vegetarian animals around the world will show you. The only problem that some vegetarians have is that there may be some amino acids missing from their diet. This can be rectified with various supplements, and is worth looking into if you are a vegetarian.

As for the amount of protein that you will need, this can and does vary according to a number of factors, including your genetics, training history, body size, and training intensity. A rough guide is to take on a gram of protein for every pound of lean body weight, or 2 grams of protein for every kilogram of bodyweight. For example, if you weigh 80 kilograms, or 160 pounds, then 160 grams of protein per day is a good target to achieve. Do not worry too much about this, as the majority of people take in sufficient protein every day to not have to count the number of grams they are eating. If you simply try and eat some protein at every meal then you will have no trouble ingesting enough into your body.

Reduce Your Carbohydrate Intake

Refined carbohydrate is one type of food that is more readily available than ever before, but causes more health problems than any other. Refined carbohydrates include white flour, white bread, pasta, white rice, sugar, and pastry, and they are bad for you for a number of reasons:

• Firstly, they have a relatively high energy density, at 4 calories per gram. This is not as high as fat, at 9 calories per gram, but people do not eat anywhere near the amount of fat as they do carbohydrates, which is the main reason why so many people have trouble with their weight.

They steer clear of fat, eating low fat yogurt, milk, cheese, etc., but think nothing of eating loaves of bread, pasta, rice, potatoes, and all manner of other starchy carbohydrates.

- Secondly, eating lots of carbohydrates can and will spike blood sugar, which can then lead to increased fat retention, blunted insulin response, and other undesirable side effects, especially to those who are training for strength and performance.

- Thirdly, many people, at least in the western world, are intolerant to some degree to yeast and gluten. Yeast and gluten especially is found in bread and most types of flour, and are often the cause of any bloated feeling you may experience from time to time. This is due to the proteins in the gluten causing inflammation in the gut, which is not a desirable situation for us, as we should be busy recovering from a strength workout, not trying to combat inflammation. If you can, research the Palaeolithic (Caveman) diet, which will tell you why it is not really a good idea for humans to eat gluten, or grains in general (see the resources section at the end of this book for further reading).

- Lastly, if you are looking to get ripped or reduce your body fat, decreasing your intake of refined carbohydrates is the best change you can make. Refined carbohydrates are very energy dense, and overeating them will contribute considerably to your level of body fat.

I completely understand that people's lives take priority, and that sometimes you will have to go out to dinner, or to parties, or to functions where you will be faced with foods that you would not eat ordinarily. This is fine, and the worst feeling is to think that all of your hard work will come undone because of one meal. If you are at a function where you cannot eat good nutritious foods, then simply try and pick your meal or the foods you eat according to the rules I have laid out in this section. For example, if the only choice is a chicken burger and fries with salad, simply ask to only have the chicken breast without the bun, leave the fries, and ask for extra salad and greens instead.

Make Food in Bulk

Anyone that has ever read any bodybuilding or muscle and fitness forums or magazines will know this rule, and that is to make food in bulk. Making food in bulk serves a number of purposes:

- Firstly, it ensures that there is always a quality meal to be eaten whenever you are hungry.

- Secondly, it enables you to take this food to work, the gym, on the train, etc., so that you do not end up buying junk food when you are away from home.

- Thirdly, it takes less time and costs less money to make food in bulk than it does to cook a separate meal every time you need to eat.

There are more than enough recipes out there to show you how to cook in bulk, so I will not bore you with any of them, but I recommend meals that have lots of nutrients. For example, I live in the UK where the weather can be cold and wet sometimes (OK, a lot of the time), so I tend to make stews, casseroles, soups and other hot meals for my bulk food. They contain plenty of protein and good fats from the meat, an abundance of carbohydrates and other nutrients from the vegetables, and they are quick and easy to eat and require no more preparation than heating up in a microwave. In addition, buying plastic tubs in which to keep the food is another very good practice. I personally have lots of these lying around, both large ones that I freeze food in, and smaller ones that I take to work, on the train, on journeys, or to the gym, etc.

Sample Diet

To finish this chapter, we will look at a sample diet that is pretty typical for me on any given day. This is only an example, and serves to show how simple, easy, and cheap it can be to eat a very good diet that will help you to build strength and athletic performance.

• Breakfast
For breakfast I almost always eat scrambled egg. This consists of 2 to 3 eggs mixed with a small amount of milk, and then cooked until ready. I often eat some fruit at the same time, most often a banana and an apple. I also pair this with plenty of water or good quality milk. Do not fall for the low fat milk fad; get the fullest fat, most nutritious stuff you can find.

• Morning Snack
For snacks I almost always eat a mixture of unprocessed nuts, seeds, and dried fruit. In my mix today are cashews, brazils, almonds, raisins, cranberries, etc. This way you eat good protein, fats, and

carbohydrates with a snack that requires no preparation. Again, fruit here is also beneficial, or even a small can of tuna or a chicken breast.

• Lunch
My lunch usually consists of a meal that I have already cooked in bulk. Examples are a tuna salad, chicken salad, beef stew, roast chicken with vegetables, etc. Make sure to have lots of vegetables along with the protein source, as this will provide plenty of nutrients that your body needs.

• Afternoon Snack
My second snack is the same as before, but can also be extra fruit or left over lunch.

• Dinner
The last meal of the day is normally another bulk meal, or can be made on the day. As an example, I may have diced chicken breast with a peanut butter and cream cheese sauce, sweet potatoes, peas, sweetcorn, asparagus, and broccoli.

Contrary to popular belief, the body does not become stronger or fitter when you are training. It becomes stronger in the intervals between training sessions, and for this to happen, it must be allowed a chance to recover. The human body is an adaptive organism, and given enough rest, the proper nutrition, and adequate sleep, it can and will recover from almost any stresses placed upon it. There are four areas that we are going to look at in this section: sleep, injury, taking care of your hands, and tendon and ligament strength.

Sleep

To recover from your workouts, there is nothing more important than adequate rest, good nutrition, and above all else, sleep. Most people, in the modern world at any rate, suffer from sleep deprivation. There is a wealth of scientific evidence to suggest that the body does not repair itself effectively if your sleep is either too short, interrupted, or if you get into bed too late. For many reasons, having a good night's sleep is something that is becoming more and more rare these days. Stress from work, a busy family life, financial worries, and many other factors can all build up to make a good night's sleep impossible. I have had these problems, and just as many of you reading this may well have done too, but there are a number of steps that you can take to ensure you get an adequate night's rest:

- Firstly, make sure that you get to bed on time. This means that you should be asleep by no later than 10:30pm: any later, and you will miss out on the valuable time necessary to allow the body to repair itself. Now I know that it is not always possible to get to bed, let alone to sleep, before 10:30pm, but on the days and nights that you can, it is important to try and do so.

- Secondly, stay off your mobile phone and any other electronic device for at least twenty minutes before you go to sleep. The bright light and glare of the screen will not be good for your eyes, and the electromagnetic field produced by these devices cannot be beneficial for your brain if it is trying to shut off at the end of the day. There is some research into this field, but as most people are more or less addicted to checking their social media profiles before turning in, not much attention has been paid to it. Ultimately, if you are serious about achieving real calisthenic strength, then your status update can wait until the morning.

- Thirdly, if there is anything that you are worrying about, such as a number of tasks you have to complete the next day, then write them down on a small notepad that you keep by the side of your bed. I started doing this a long time ago and it helps immensely. If like me you have thousands of thoughts and ideas bouncing around, then write them down. I have found that this almost locks them away in a sense, so that my mind can clear and I always sleep better because of it.

- Fourthly, make your bedroom as dark as possible. This is a no-brainer, as the darker the room the easier it will be for you to shut off and get to sleep more quickly. Try getting dark shaded curtains or draping a towel or similar over the existing curtains or blinds.

- Lastly, try and learn to meditate. Now, I am not a spiritualist and do not believe in any new age philosophy, but the ability to shut out thoughts and relax the brain is very rare in the modern world, and can be enormously useful to those of you who still struggle to sleep even after following all of the steps mentioned above.

What To Do If You Are Injured

Although there is little chance of getting injured when performing calisthenics, nevertheless the more advanced exercises do place a large amount of stress and strain on the bones, muscles, tendons, and ligaments of the body, so the chance and risk of injury is never completely zero. There are steps you can take to avoid becoming injured, like not overtraining, only progressing when you are ready, and above all else, allowing enough time for your body to adapt to the demands being placed upon it. Also, make sure to follow the mobility and flexibility drills that are explained and demonstrated in Chapter 4, as this will help to correct and prevent any issues arising in the future. If you do become injured, then the best response is to rest and seek professional advice, preferably from a reputable physiotherapist with knowledge of sports and strength training injuries. The most common niggles and injuries you may come across in your own training are unique to calisthenics, and it is worth talking about a few of them here, just so you know what to look out for, and what to do if you succumb to them.

- As the elbow joint is used extensively in calisthenics, there is a slight risk of tendonitis. Planches, front levers, back levers, and human flags are all performed with straight arms and, whilst this is not harmful, overuse can occur and the elbow joint can become quite sore and inflexible. The same will happen when training for one-arm pull-ups and the other movements that place a lot of strain on the ligaments and tendons of the upper body joints. As I explain in the exercise section, this is why I recommend keeping the repetition ranges low on movements like the one-arm pull-up and other similar exercises.

- The core takes a huge pounding in nearly all calisthenic exercises, so watch out for soreness and any stresses and strains in this area. A couple of times in my own training I have overdone it and pulled my abs, so much so that it was difficult to get out of bed for a week or so. If this is the case, then again, more rest and less training time will be the solution. Any serious injury, like a hernia, needs to be treated and seen by a qualified medical professional.

- The shoulders probably come under the most stress during calisthenic training. That is because, as I explained in Chapter 1, the scapulae are, by definition, the most unstable joints in the body. This means that the chance of injury here is higher than in many other parts of the body and adequate warm-ups and mobility exercises are essential. In Chapter 4, you will be exposed to scapula-strengthening movements that can help to build almost bombproof shoulders. If you are serious about training for a long time and do not want to become injured, please ensure that you adhere to them.

- Lastly, the hands will be involved in almost all of the exercises that are featured in this book and in all calisthenic movements, and as such, will be placed under enormous stress and strain every time you workout. Make sure that you stretch them before and after each session, and if you feel any unusual pain in them whatsoever, cease the exercise and rest.

Taking Care of Your Hands

As I have already explained, out of all of the parts of the body involved in calisthenics, the one that is used the most is undoubtedly the hands. For almost every exercise, including pushing, pulling, and many of the core exercises, the hands are used extensively and can really take a beating, so it is important that we look after them. In the same way that we perform mobility and strengthening exercises for the shoulders, and perform flexibility drills for the whole body, we should look after the hands.

- When you start calisthenic training, you may notice that the palms of the hands can be quite sore, especially after a heavy pull-up session, or after using parallettes for an extended period of time. This is a normal and natural reaction on the body's part, so you should not attempt to inhibit the soreness, except rest and maybe moisturise. Do *not* be tempted to start using gloves. This will only cause more problems later on, especially when you begin to learn the false grip and other movements that require complete feel and sensitivity in the hands.

- The second change that will happen, in response to the soreness and the use of the hands, is that the body will form calluses, most commonly where the fingers join the palm and on each joint of the fingers themselves. This is again normal, but you should not allow them to become too big, as these often have the negative effect of getting caught on things, and of getting in the way when grabbing a pull-up bar or other object. They will also bunch up and squash whenever the hand is closed into a fist, which again can be uncomfortable. The best solution that I have found is to sand down and reduce the height of the calluses to the point that they are still there, but not gone entirely. You can use a number of tools for this job, like nail files, very light sandpaper, and certain beauty products designed for getting rid of dry and dead skin. This is important for a number of reasons, the main one being that the skin hardens in those places for a reason, and that you need this to stop blisters and other rips and tears from happening. It may seem big and clever to have torn hands, and not a week goes by where I do not see a picture of someone's bleeding hands posted proudly on the Internet, but the most this will do is just give you a few weeks off training, which is not an ideal situation if you are trying to progress and become stronger.

- Lastly, if you use some form of chalk in your training, and especially if you use liquid chalk, then your hands will definitely need moisturiser applied to them after every workout. The alcohol in liquid chalk will dry out your hands completely, leaving them more prone to damage from rips and tears, so make sure that you do this, no matter how un-macho it may seem. It is much more un-macho to have to take time away from training because you did not take two minutes to look after your hands.

Tendon and Ligament Strength

The last part of this section deals with tendon and ligament strength, and the ways in which it differs from muscular strength.

Whilst muscles are responsible for moving the joints and therefore for all of human movement, the tendons connect muscles to bone, and the ligaments connect bone to bone. An often neglected or misunderstood part of strength training, is that all parts of the body take the same time to heal and recover. This is not true, and in our case it is particularly important, as calisthenic training relies heavily on the strength of the tendons and ligaments. If we take the example of the planche, there is a huge amount of force that must be transferred through the biceps tendon and the other connective tissues in order for the movement to be completed. If you do not allow adequate time for these tissues to heal, then you will not recover in time, and you will not become stronger.

Estimates vary, but for the average person, tendons and ligaments take up to ten times as long to heal if they are injured than the muscles that surround them. This means that if muscles take three days to heal from a strain, then the tendon or ligament will take thirty days to heal from a strain/ sprain. If you feel pain in the elbows or any other area not associated with muscular soreness, then rest. Do not be tempted to push your luck: you will injure yourself even more and may set yourself back weeks or months.

Physical Preparation

In this section we are going to look at a number of very important parts of training that are often overlooked completely by many people. These are warming up, mobility, exercise preparation, and flexibility. All of these stages are vital if you wish to progress quickly and without injury, and I would encourage you to read and absorb as much as possible.

Warming Up

Warming up before any exercise is a good idea, but it becomes even more important if you are going to train using calisthenics. The amount of muscle used and the intensity of those muscle contractions make it essential that you are fully warmed up and prepared before starting a workout. This is not to say you must spend hours going through every warm up exercise known to man. In my experience some people spend far too long warming up, at the expense of actually training, and see poor results because they simply do not spend enough time actually performing the movements that contribute towards strength gains. In addition, if you spend too long or expend too much effort warming up there is a chance you will not be able to put as much effort into your actual workout. This is a big mistake, as you need to try and gain as much out of each session as possible.

The first part of your warm-up needs to be cardiovascular, to elevate the body temperature and to make the muscles, tendons, and ligaments warm and supple. This can be anything that you like, but there are a certain number of activities that work better than others. Running or jogging is the easiest, as it does not require any equipment and can be carried out even in a relatively small space. If you have access to a gym, then the cardiovascular machines are very good for the initial warm-up. The bike, rowing machine, and cross trainer or elliptical are all good pieces of equipment for raising the body temperature and increasing the heart rate. The amount of time that you will have to do this for depends entirely on the person,

but 5 to 8 minutes is normally long enough for the majority of people to feel warm and ready for their workout. Whichever method you choose, as long as you feel physically and mentally ready for the workout at the end of it, then that is adequate.

Mobility

Once you have warmed up to a good level, it is recommended you engage in some mobility work prior to actually starting your full workout. Mobility can be roughly defined as the body's ability to move into positions under the muscles' own power. Lack of mobility can seriously hinder your progress, as not being able to get into the correct body positions will not allow you to exert as much force in the exercise and will limit your strength gains.

Mobility itself has become far more common and widespread in the years that I have been studying training methods and programming, and it is very rare nowadays to find any athlete that either does not mobilise or does not think of it as beneficial. It can also help to alleviate pain and soreness in the muscles, eradicate any knots and tight areas, and just keep everything working properly.

I have broken down the mobility exercises into three parts: upper body mobility, core or torso mobility, and lower body mobility. Ideally these exercises should be performed at the start of every workout, but this is not absolutely essential. Mobility is one of those strange activities that the more you do the less you need to do. This may seem counterintuitive, but once you have good mobility, you will have to spend far less time maintaining it than you did acquiring it in the first place.

For some of the mobility movements you will simply need to get into a certain body position, or move into a certain position and out of it again, but for others you will need access to a foam roller, as described in the equipment section.

Upper Body Mobility

Upper body mobility is often neglected in preference to spending time on the lower body, especially the hamstrings. The hamstrings are tight in most people, which is maybe why so much time is spent stretching them. Yet upper body flexibility and mobility, particularly in the shoulder girdle, is very important in order to be able to transfer power and deal with physical situations that arise in any sport. Poor upper body mobility will also prevent you from getting into positions such as the handstand, and will only hinder you in the long run.

The first few mobility exercises that we are going to look at are the scapula push-up, scapula dip, scapula pull-up, and scapula one-armed pull-up. These exercises are designed to strengthen and increase the mobility of the whole shoulder girdle, and have long been a staple of my training.

Scapula Push-ups

This is an invaluable exercise that can be very useful when preparing for the planche and some of the other levers, such as the front lever and back lever. It can be thought of as a 'pushing' scapula exercise, and again is useful in floor movements such as the planche and various levers.

1. Position yourself in a push-up position with a neutral stance.

2. From here, lower your chest down to the floor, squeezing your scapula together as you do so. Do *not* bend the elbows.

3. Once you reach the bottom position, reverse the movement so that your shoulder blades separate and your spine rises up. Keep pushing until your back rounds and your spine is as elevated as possible. Do *not* bend the elbows at any point during the movement. Repeat for 10 repetitions.

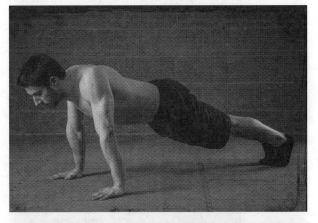

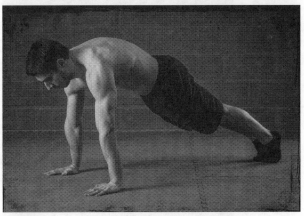

Scapula Dip

The second scapula pushing exercise is the scapula dip. (This should really be called the reverse scapula shrug as it is the opposite movement to a traditional shrug.) It is designed to strengthen the shoulders for movements such as handstands, planches, and other floor-based exercises.

1. Position yourself in the top part of a triceps dip. Keep the body neutral.

2. From here, allow your whole body to sink, so that your shoulders rise up to meet your ears. Keep your elbows locked throughout.

3. From this bottom position, push up hard, aiming to move the whole body into the air and the shoulders down as far as possible. Do *not* bend your elbows at any point. Repeat for 10 repetitions.

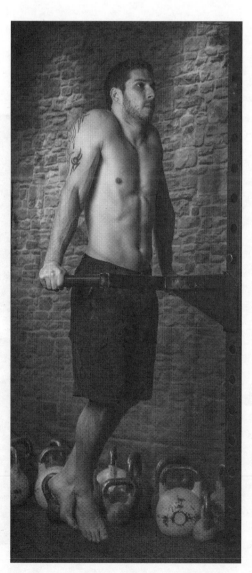 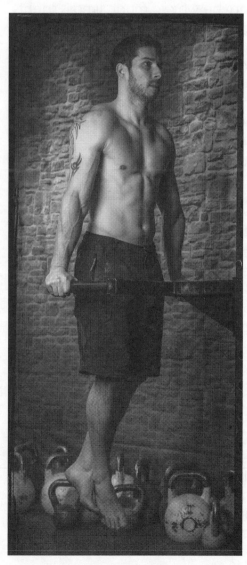

Scapula Pull-up

One of the most useful exercises we can use to develop scapula strength is what I call the scapula pull-up. These develop a huge amount of strength as you are effectively working with your entire bodyweight.

1. Grab a pull-up bar with an overhand grip and hang with completely straight arms.

2. Make sure that your scapulae are elevated, so that your shoulders are close to or touching your ears.

3. From this dead hang position, attempt to pull your scapulae down *without* bending your elbows. At first this may feel impossible to master, but persevere until you can. The range of motion you will achieve depends on a number of factors, including your strength, flexibility, and shoulder physiology.

4. Once you have pulled your scapulae down, hold this position for a second, then drop back down to the start position. Repeat for 10 repetitions. You can also use weight with this exercise to great effect.

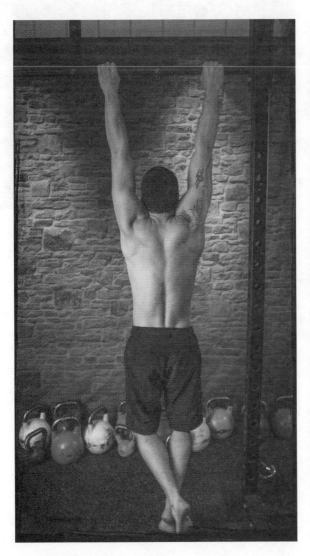
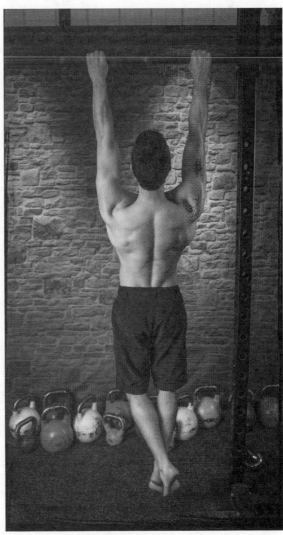

Scapula One-Arm Pull-up

Once you have become familiar with the scapula pull-up, you can move onto the one-armed version. This variation will be invaluable in learning one-arm pull-ups, as one of the most difficult parts of the one-arm pull-up (if not *the* most difficult), is starting the pull from the dead hang position. This part becomes much easier as your scapulae increase in strength.

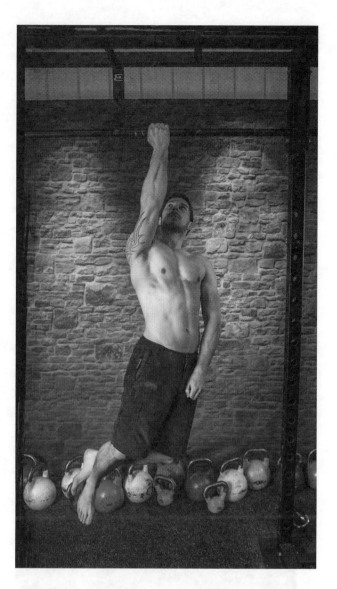

1. Grab a pull-up bar with one hand in an overhand or underhand grip and hang with a completely locked arm. You can put the other arm wherever you like, but I prefer to have it crossed over my chest or in front of my torso.

2. Make sure that your scapula is elevated, so that your shoulder is close to or touching your ear.

3. From this dead hang position, attempt to pull your scapula down, *without* bending your elbow. At first this may feel impossible to master, but persevere until you can. The range of motion you will achieve depends on a number of factors, including your strength, flexibility, and shoulder physiology.

4. Once you have pulled your scapula down, hold this position for a few seconds, then drop back down to the start position. Repeat for 5 repetitions on each arm.

Scapula Foam Rolling

As well as actually exercising and strengthening the scapulae, it is important to foam roll them, particularly if you have any tight or sore areas or knots within the muscle. This can help greatly to increase mobility in this area.

1. Position yourself on top of the foam roller, and then put your body into a hollow position. To do this, hug yourself so that your back rounds.

2. Now roll backwards and forwards over the foam roller, stopping and going slower when you hit any sore points. Spend about twenty to thirty seconds doing this.

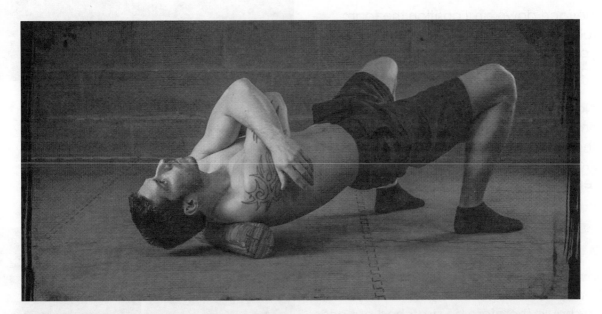

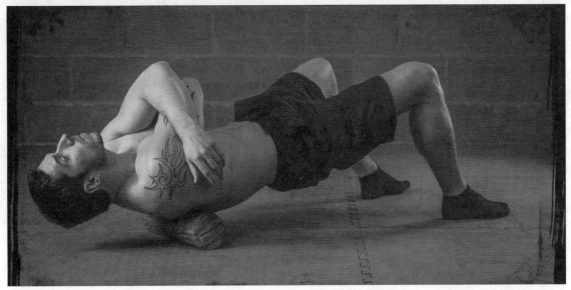

Armpit Foam Rolling

Most people are tight in the chest and armpits. This is a consequence of the modern world, where many people spend hours every day either sitting at a desk or driving. This causes the muscles in the front of the body to shorten and tighten, and those in the back to stretch and become weaker. We can correct this by foam rolling certain areas, and for this mobility drill we are going to foam roll the armpit.

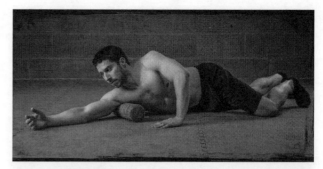

1. Lie face down and position the foam roller at 90-degrees to the body. Extend your arm up over your head and position your armpit right on top of the roller.

2. Now roll forwards and backwards ten times, taking care to move slower over the sore parts and allow the roller do its work. Then move to the other side and repeat.

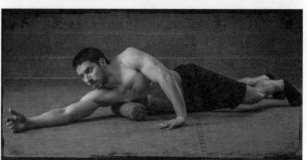

Rotator Cuff Stretch

The rotator cuff musculature is responsible for much of the movement of the shoulder, and should therefore be stretched out prior to any exercise involving the shoulders.

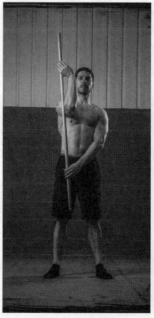
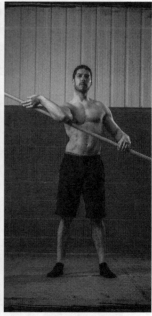

1. Grab a bar or pole and hold it as shown. It should be pressed onto the outside of your upper arm.

2. From here, push the bar up towards the ceiling. You should feel a big stretch in the rotator cuff musculature. Hold this for ten seconds, then switch arms and repeat.

Chest and Shoulder Stretch

Opening up the chest and shoulders is very important before embarking on a training session. This next stretch is one of most effective for stretching and mobilising the shoulders, armpits, and chest.

1. Find a space on the ground and get onto your hands and knees.

2. Now push your hips into the air and move your chest towards the ground. Keep thinking of pulling the shoulders and chest down through the ground to increase the stretch. Hold this for around 15 to 20 seconds and release.

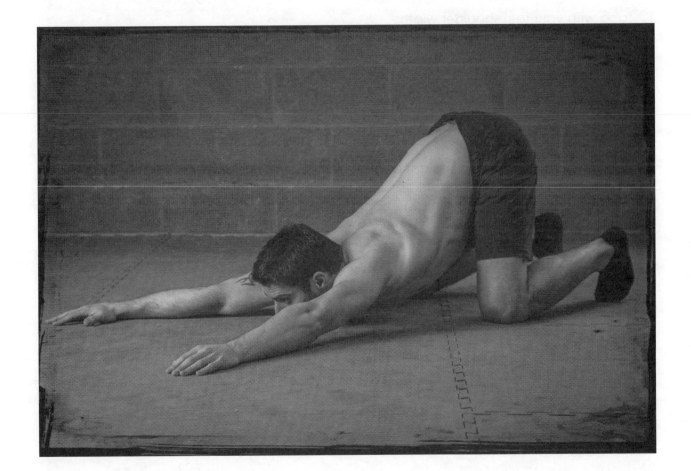

Shoulder Dislocates

The last of our upper body mobility drills are shoulder dislocates. Don't worry, your shoulders won't actually dislocate, but if you have tight shoulders or poor upper body flexibility, you will really feel these. To perform them you will need a bar or pole, preferably one that is very light. Broom handles or exercise class barbells are excellent for this movement.

1. Stand with your feet shoulder width apart, and hold the bar in front of you with an overhand grip. Start with as wide a grip as you can manage.

2. From here, move the bar up over the head in a large arc, finishing with the bar resting on your lower back. Ensure that you keep your elbows straight at all times. Perform 2 sets of 10 repetitions with around 20 to 30 seconds rest in between each set.

Teaching Points

If you struggle to perform the movement at all, try moving the hands further apart until you can. As your shoulders become more flexible, simply move the hands closer together to increase the difficulty of the movement. The following pictures show the movement in full.

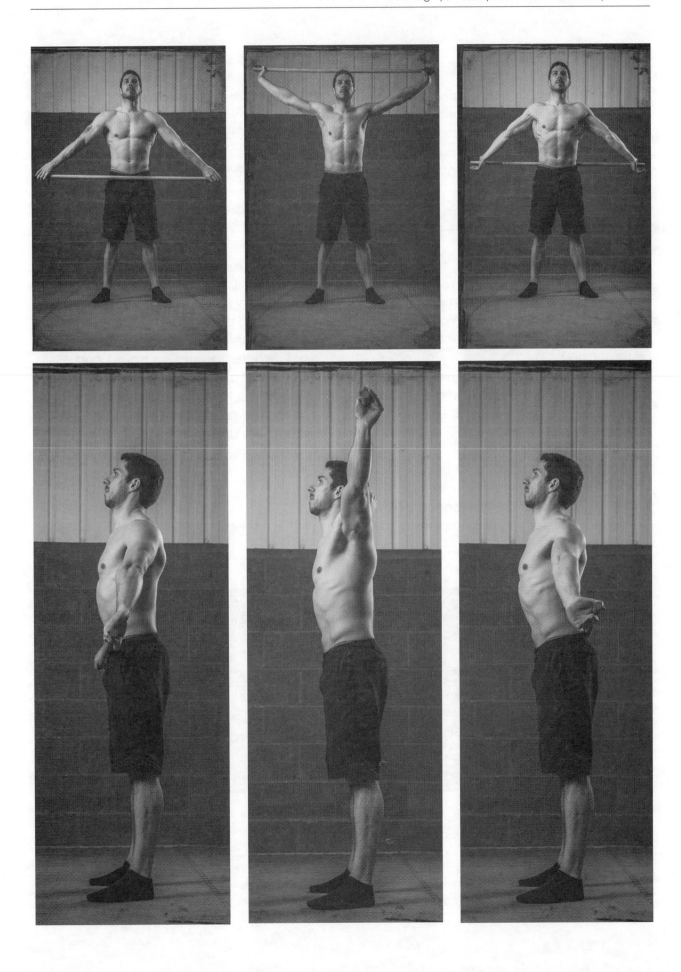

Core Mobility

Core mobility is a little less comprehensive than the upper body or lower body mobility, because the core cannot move as much as the upper body and lower body, and the spine is incapable of a wide range of movements. However, it is still important for you to keep and maintain core mobility, as you do not want to be limited in your movements by lack of flexibility in the spine.

Spine Foam Rolling

As described earlier, foam rolling is an invaluable addition to a mobility routine, and can help to alleviate some injury problems or lack of mobility. Foam rolling the spine is good for a couple of reasons. Firstly, it can help to reduce the number of knots and tight areas within particular muscle groups in the back, and secondly, it can improve the ability of the spine to extend.

1. Position a foam roller at 90-degrees to your torso and place your lower back on it. Keep your feet on the floor and have your hands ready to help support you if you need it.

2. Starting at the base of the spine, roll backwards and forwards along the roller, slowing down on any sore parts and paying particular attention to them. Continue until you reach the top of the back, where you should pause and allow your spine to curl around the roller. This will help to stretch the chest and encourage greater mobility and flexibility around the upper back.

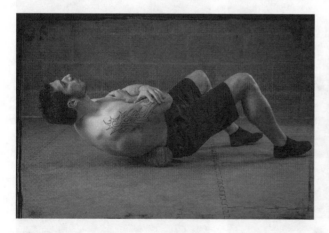
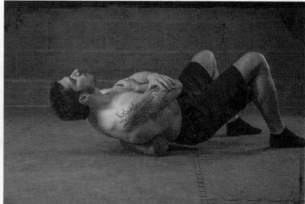

Side Leans

One part of the core that is particularly troublesome for many people is the obliques. These are the muscles in the sides of the torso and are responsible for allowing you to bend sideways at the waist. The lower part of your spine will also dictate how flexible you will be here, so this exercise is also important for those of you who have a low level of spinal flexibility. To perform side leans, you will need a bar or pole, preferably the same type that you used for the shoulder dislocates.

1. Stand with your feet wide apart and grasp a bar with both hands, with your hands approximately as wide as your feet, so that your entire body forms a large "X" shape.

2. From here, bend over to one side at the waist, using the muscles in the sides of your core. Keep your arms straight at all times and do not allow your shoulders to move towards your head; the movement must only come from your waist.

3. Once you have gone as low as possible, return to the upright position and repeat on the other side. Repeat for 10 repetitions.

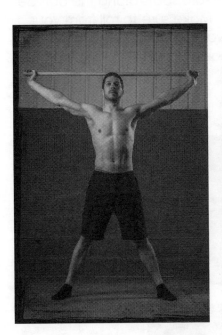 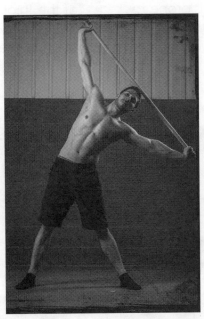 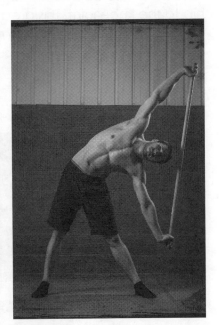

Lower Body Mobility

The lower body is used continuously as a method of transportation during everyday life, so even if you don't train or take part in any sporting activity, it is often home to many mobility problems. Usually this manifests itself in mobility and performance issues later on, and can be troublesome to correct once it reaches that stage. Thankfully, improving and maintaining lower body mobility is very straightforward. The exercises and mobility drills that I have presented in this next section can be utilised daily for optimum results, ideally before your training begins, and even on rest days to keep everything moving properly. The actual movements themselves are based around stretches and foam rolling movements that have long been part of strength and conditioning programs, with extra input from Joe DeFranco from DeFranco's gym in the United States. There are many different exercises that you can perform for mobility, but the ones presented here are those that I have found to be the most effective and that I use on a very regular basis.

IT Band Foam Rolling

The first part of our lower body preparation is to foam roll the IT band. The proper name for this part of the anatomy is the iliotibial band (or tract), which is a long tendon that runs down the outside of the thigh from the hip to the knee joint. This area is prone to being overtight, especially in runners, and can cause numerous knee issues.

1. Lie down on one side with the outside of your thigh resting on a roller.

2. Now roll backwards and forwards until you find any sore spots along the outside of the thigh. Make sure to roll from your hip all the way down to the knee joint. Spend at least 15 seconds rolling on each leg.

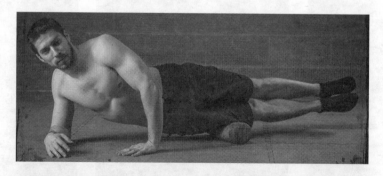

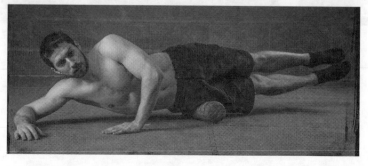

Adductor Foam Rolling

Together with the hamstrings and the glutes, the adductors play their part in hip drive and the production of power throughout the lower body, so it is important that they remain mobile and unrestricted.

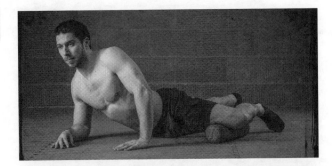

1. Place the foam roller on the ground at 90 degrees to your body, placing the inside of the thigh against it.

2. Now roll sideways from the inside of the knee into the hip itself. Spend at least 15 seconds rolling on each leg.

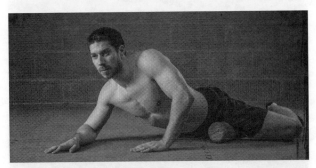

Piriformis Foam Rolling

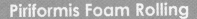

As you start to incorporate more squatting and hip movements into your training, you may find that the piriformis, or the muscle on the outside of the hip, becomes overtight. The best way to counteract this is to roll the piriformis. You can either use a foam roller as I have done here, or you can use a ball, e.g. a tennis ball.

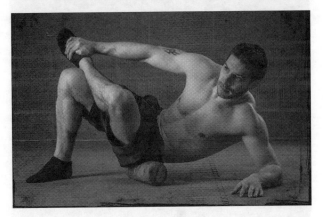

1. Sit down and place your right foot on the left knee, as if you were going to cross your legs.

2. Now sit directly on the foam roller or ball with the piriformis. You will know if you are on the right spot because it will feel sore. Roll over the tight or tender spot slowly, or simply sit on the spot and allow the ball or roller to sink into the muscle, making sure to spend the most time on the area that is the sorest. Then change legs and repeat.

Static Stretch

Once you have rolled the piriformis, you should perform a static stretch.

1. Sit on a bench with your right foot flat on the floor and the knee at 90 degrees.

2. Place your left foot over the knee of the right leg and push down on the left knee. You will feel the stretch in the side of the glute. Try and keep the torso upright and breathe deeply. Hold the stretch for 15 seconds and then change sides and repeat.

Rollovers into Straddle Sit

Rollovers generate mobility and flexibility in many areas of the lower body, including the glutes, hamstrings, groin, and the hip area in general. This exercise requires a bit of flexibility in the hips, so just do as much as you can.

1. Sit down with your legs in front of you.

2. Now roll backwards onto your back and throw your legs behind your head.

3. Push yourself forwards to a seated position again, but spread your legs into a wide straddle position. As you do this, reach forwards between your legs as far as possible. This counts as one repetition. Perform 10 repetitions of this exercise.

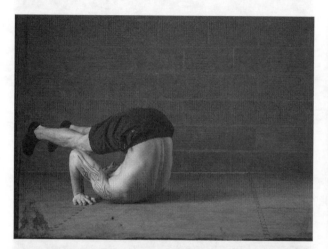
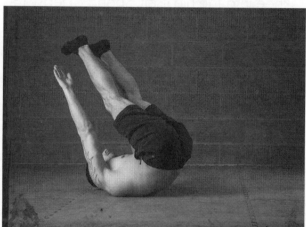
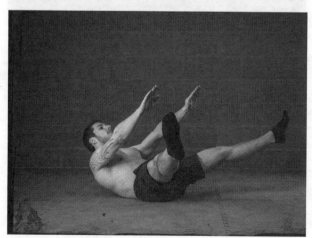
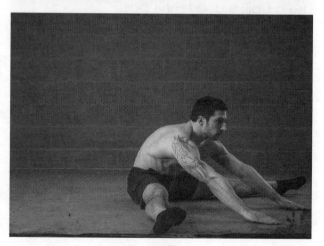

Knee Circles

Knee circles are another really great lower body mobility exercise that help to open up the hips in preparation for the lower body movements.

1. Position yourself on your hands and knees.

2. From here, raise one leg up to the side, extend the knee backwards and then bring it forwards as far as you can before placing it down on the floor again. The aim of this exercise is to draw a very large arc with the knee. Perform the movement 10 times forwards and 10 times backwards on each leg.

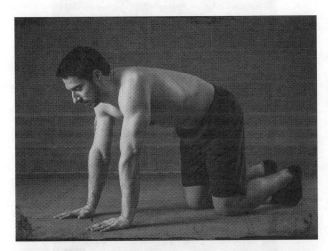
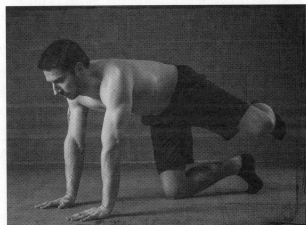
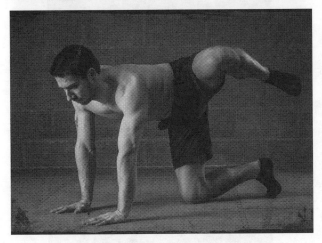
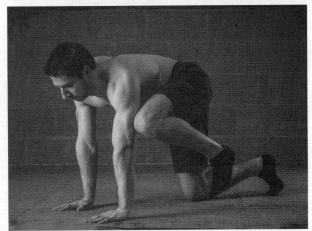

Mountain Climbers

Mountain climbers are an awesome conditioning and metabolism-raising exercise and with a small alteration they can also help to create more mobility in the hips. You will also get a good hip flexor and hamstring stretch in this exercise.

1. Get into a push-up position with one leg stretched out behind you and the other placed as close to the side of your hand as possible.

2. Keeping your arms straight, jump both feet into the air and change them over, so that the rear foot comes to the front and the front foot goes to the rear. Repeat for 10 repetitions.

Frog Hops

Frog hops are a variation of mountain climbers that require more flexibility because both feet will be moving to the sides of the hands. Make sure that you jump with both feet out wide so that your legs do not knock into your arms.

1. Get into a push-up position.

2. From here, jump both feet forwards until they reach the outside of your hands, then jump them back so that you reach the push-up position again. This requires good hip mobility so just keep working with them until you can reach the position shown in the pictures. Perform 10 repetitions.

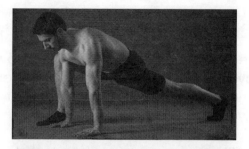
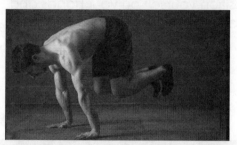
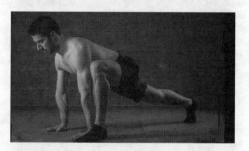
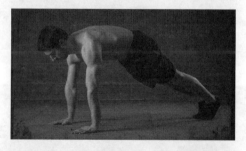
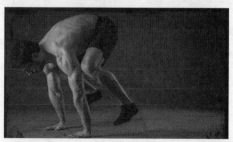
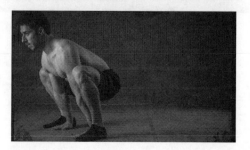

Hip Flexor Stretch

Tight hip flexors are responsible for many performance issues, including inadequate hip drive and power, and can also pull the pelvis into awkward positions that are not ideal for athletes. Stretching them is therefore a vital part of your physical preparation. This stretch is the same as the one in the flexibility section (see page 69).

1. Place one knee on the floor and the other foot in front. Both knees should be at 90 degrees.

2. Now lean forwards until you begin to feel a stretch in the front of the hip of the rear leg. Aim to keep your torso upright at all times. If you do not feel the stretch, increase the distance between your foot and knee. Repeat the stretch for 10 seconds on each leg.

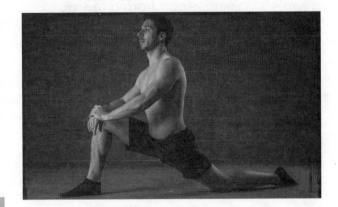

Deep Squat Position

In addition to all of the other mobility exercises we have looked at so far, this one is perhaps the most effective of the lot. Simply sitting in the deep squat position will correct most of your lower body mobility problems. In the Western world, nearly all adults and many children have lost this ability due to their inactive lifestyle, but in other cultures, this skill is routinely practiced.

The best time to do these are when you are relaxing, e.g. when you are either watching television or reading, etc. This ensures that it becomes part of your regular routine and you will soon see your mobility quickly improve.

1. Place your heels shoulder width apart and point your toes slightly out.

2. Bend your knees, push your hips back, and squat down as far as you can. Keep your lower back as straight as possible.

3. Once you are as low as possible, place your elbows on the insides of your knees and push them out slightly. Remain in this position for as long as possible, aiming for a total time of 5 minutes or more. Note below the position you should be striving to attain.

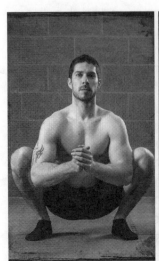
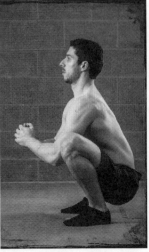

Flexibility

Having looked at a number of mobility exercises, we now turn our attention to flexibility. Flexibility is the ability of your muscles to allow your joints to move in any direction without restriction, and for calisthenics the biggest problem areas are the shoulders and hips. Flexibility is probably the most neglected part of most people's training. Apart from a few quick stretches after their workout, most people never spend any time trying to improve their flexibility. It is important for injury prevention, maintaining mobility (especially as we get older), improving recovery rates, and performing some of the more difficult exercises in this book. Although a complete guide to flexibility is outside the scope of this volume, the stretches I have included still have many benefits. If you wish to learn more about flexibility, then there are many good books on the subject, with my preferred choice being *Relax into Stretch* by Pavel Tsatsouline (see the resources section at the end of this book).

In these days of driving, computers and office work, most people's upper bodies are unbalanced with tight muscles in the front of the body and weak and loose muscles in the back. This can easily be demonstrated in the posture of many people, who may have rounded shoulders, a forwards jutting head, and an inability to raise their arms above their head. Correcting this problem takes a little time but is well worth the effort.

The lower body also contains numerous problems for many people. The hips can be thought of as the hinge of the body, and if the areas around the hips are not flexible, then you will have real trouble with some of the exercises in this book. Lack of flexibility in this area can be due to a number of factors, but more often

than not it is as a result of tightness in the hamstrings, adductors or groin, and the piriformis. Luckily, these problems are easily addressed, and once you have acquired the level of flexibility and mobility you need, it can be maintained with very little effort.

A common misconception about flexibility is that it is controlled by the physical shortness of your muscles. This is untrue. Flexibility, or the ability of your muscles to lengthen, is controlled by your nervous system, and is not due to your muscles actually "stretching". When you reach the limit of your flexibility it is the *stretch reflex* firing that stops you going further. To become more flexible, you need to re-educate your nervous system to allow your muscles to achieve their full length. There are many ways that you can do this, but I have picked three of the best and outlined them below.

• Relax

You must be relaxed for your flexibility to improve, so avoid being too tense, anxious, or uncomfortable. There are many ways to promote relaxation, but one of the easiest and best methods is to contrast your breathing.

To do this, choose a stretch, and then increase it until you reach your limit. Hold this for 10 seconds or so before taking a deep in-breath. Hold this breath for a couple of seconds and then release it all in one go. As you do so, attempt to make your whole body relax. Your stretch should increase. Repeat this process 3 to 5 times.

• Make a lengthened muscle stronger

Perhaps the best way to improve your flexibility is to increase the strength of the muscle you are stretching, whilst in a stretched position. If a muscle is stronger in a lengthened position, the nervous system is much more likely to allow the body to get into that position in the first place.

To increase the strength of a stretched muscle, simply assume a stretch position of your choice. From here, contract the stretched muscle whilst staying in the stretched position. Hold the contraction for 5 to 10 seconds before relaxing and increasing the stretch. This can be repeated 2 to 3 times before most people reach their limit. For the best results, you can combine the two methods above to considerably increase your flexibility.

• Be consistent

Like anything in life, it is much better to stretch for 10 minutes daily than 2 hours once a month. Consistency will help to reinforce and re-educate your nervous system into allowing you to become more flexible.

Stretching Schedule

Initially you will want to stretch after every workout. This stops the muscles becoming too tight and maintains the mobility that you have acquired. In order to significantly increase your flexibility, you will need to dedicate some time just to stretching. For most beginners, a heavy stretching session of 20 to 30 minutes once a week is more than adequate. You will probably feel quite sore afterwards, but this is normal. You can steadily increase the number of stretching sessions you perform in a week as you become more flexible and as your body learns to cope with the demands you place on it. If you feel stiff and sore the majority of the time, then you are stretching too hard or too often. If this happens, just reduce the intensity or amount of stretching that you do.

After a while you will no doubt reach the level of flexibility that you desire or need for performing your preferred exercises. When this happens, you can stop trying to increase your flexibility further and just concentrate on maintaining your current level of flexibility. The amount of stretching time required to maintain this level varies from person to person, so you will just have to experiment and find out. Most commonly, maintaining your flexibility takes far less time than actually becoming flexible in the first place.

Upper Body Stretches

The upper body is an important part of calisthenics and is used in most of the exercises that are defined as calisthenic. For this reason, stretching the upper body is a vital part of your training. These stretches are to be undertaken after your workout, but can be carried out before or during your session if you feel tight in a particular area, or feel that you need a little more mobility before a specific exercise.

Chest and Shoulder Stretch

The first stretch in this section is both a shoulder and a chest stretch, and is exactly the same as the one we looked at in the mobility section (see page 49).

1. Find a space on the ground and get onto your hands and knees.

2. Now push your hips into the air and move your chest towards the ground. Keep thinking of pulling the shoulders and chest down through the ground to increase the stretch. Hold this for around 15 to 20 seconds and release.

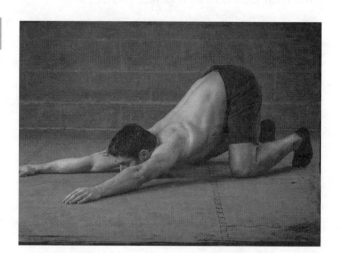

Upper Back Stretch

Once you reach the more difficult pulling exercises, your back will be under a lot of stress, so it is important to stretch your upper back to avoid any problems that may result. This particular stretch places great emphasis on the latissimus dorsi, or the big wing-like muscles on the back.

1. To perform this stretch, grasp a solid object with one arm and lean back, keeping your arm and legs straight.

2. Open up your shoulder blades and squeeze your shoulders together in front of you. Reach your opposite arm through the gap to increase the stretch. Hold this position for 15 to 20 seconds.

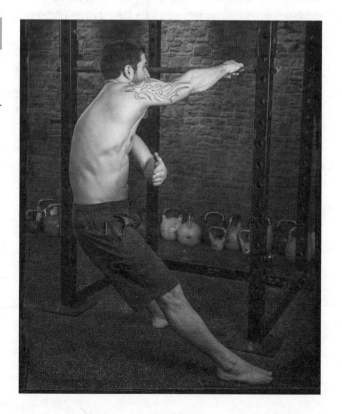

Chest Stretch

As many calisthenic exercises use a "hollow body" position where the shoulders are rounded and the chest is tensed, it is important to stretch your chest to prevent you from becoming overtight.

1. Place your palms against a solid object such as a wall or doorframe. Here I am using a squat rack. You can also perform this stretch using a single arm only.

2. Keeping your arms straight, lean forwards until you feel the stretch. Hold this position for 15 seconds, switch sides and repeat.

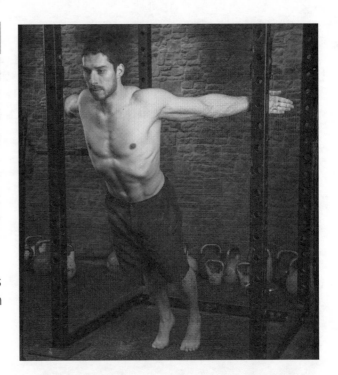

Forearm and Wrist Stretch 1

Many of the handstand and pressing exercises are extremely taxing on the wrists, so you may wish to stretch them out prior to, and after, your workout. There are two main wrist stretches. This is the first.

1. Position yourself on your hands and knees and place your hands with your fingers facing forwards.

2. Keeping your arms straight, lean forwards and attempt to keep your palms pressed into the ground. Hold this position for 15 seconds.

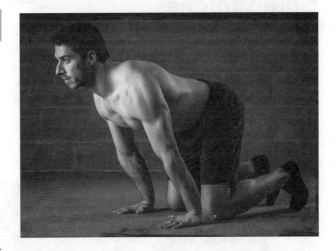

Forearm and Wrist Stretch 2

The second wrist stretch targets the upper side of the forearm, and is particularly useful after handstands and other similar exercises.

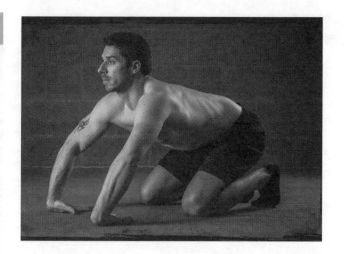

1. Position yourself on your hands and knees and place your hands on the ground with your palms facing up.

2. Point your fingers back towards your body, and keeping your arms straight, pull your body backwards until you feel the stretch. Hold for 15 seconds.

Core Stretches

It is not only in the core exercises where the core muscles are used, but also in the upper body movements, e.g. the front lever and the pull-up. This means that stretching the core is pretty important if you want to remain mobile and flexible throughout the spine. As the core muscles are not that flexible however, and as the torso is not capable of as great a range of movement as other parts of the body, range of motion will always be somewhat limited.

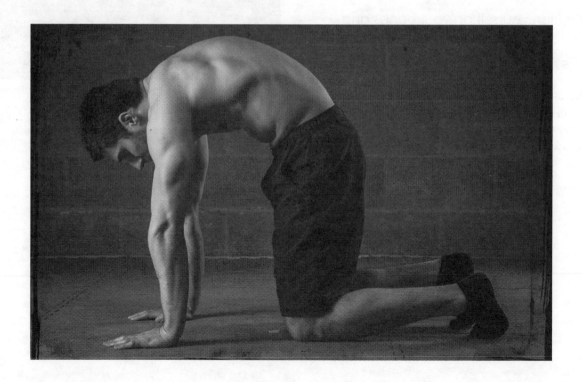

Standing Side Stretch

It is important to maintain mobility in the sides of your torso to allow you to perform the exercises that require flexibility in the spine. We can use the stretch that we looked at earlier for this purpose. To perform the standing side stretch you will need a bar or pole, preferably the same type that you used for the shoulder dislocates.

1. Stand with your feet wide apart and grasp the bar with both hands above your head, with your hands approximately as wide as your feet, so that your entire body forms a large "X" shape.

2. From here, bend over to one side at the waist, using the muscles in the sides of your core. Keep your arms straight at all times and do not allow your shoulders to move towards your head. The movement must only come from your waist.

3. Once you have reached over as low as possible, hold for 10 seconds, then switch to the other side and repeat for another 10 seconds.

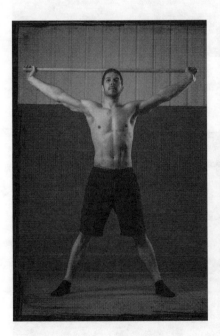
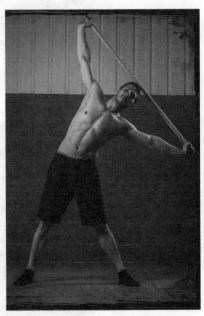
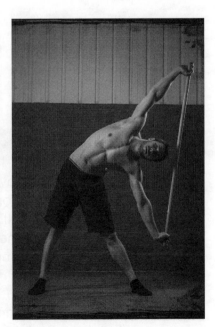

Cobra Stretch

A well-known yoga pose, the cobra stretch is good for the rectus abdominis, or six-pack, and will help to alleviate cramp or soreness after dishes, half levers, and other core exercises.

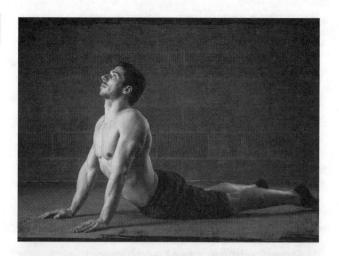

1. Lie face down with your hands flat on the floor. Push up with your arms, keeping your hips in contact with the ground.

2. Curl your spine and look up at the ceiling until you feel the stretch. Breathing deeply in and out can help to increase the stretch in this position. Hold for 15 seconds.

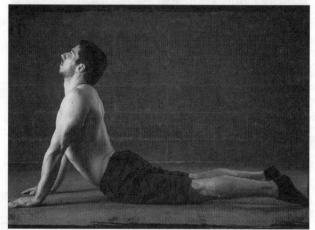

Cat Stretch

The cat stretch is another movement taken from yoga, and is excellent for targeting the middle and lower back. It will also help to teach the separation of the shoulder blades that is needed for some of the other strength exercises.

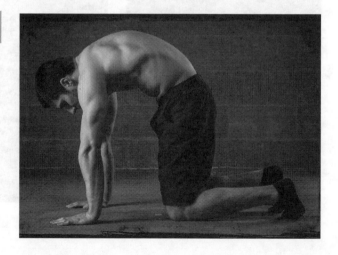

1. Position yourself on your hands and knees and push your spine up towards the ceiling.

2. Squeeze your chest together and attempt to pull your shoulder blades apart. Hold for 15 seconds.

Lower Body Stretches

In this section we will look at the stretches that can be used to increase the flexibility of the lower body. Flexibility and mobility in the lower body is very important, and it is very easy to lose this function as you become older. It can also help you to perform the movements in the exercise section more easily. For example, performing a movement like a straddle planche becomes much easier if you build flexibility in the hips. This will allow you to increase your straddle, improving your ability to hold the planche position, thus making your progress more rapid.

Quad Stretch

The quads, or the front of the upper leg, are involved in nearly all lower body movements, and so stretching them is vital to keep proper function in the lower body.

1. Lie down on the ground as shown below.

2. Grasp one foot and pull your heel towards your butt. Ensure your knees are close together and push your hips forwards. Hold this position for 15 seconds, change sides and repeat.

Hamstring Stretch

The hamstrings, or the backs of the upper leg, are again involved in nearly all lower body movements, and are particularly susceptible to being tight in the vast majority of people. Therefore, you may want to spend longer stretching them than other muscle groups.

1. Sit down and stretch one leg out in front of you, keeping your toes pointing towards the ceiling.

2. Tuck your other foot into the side of your leg and reach forwards with your arm and try to touch your toes. Try and keep your back straight and fold from the hips. Hold this position for 15 seconds, change sides and repeat.

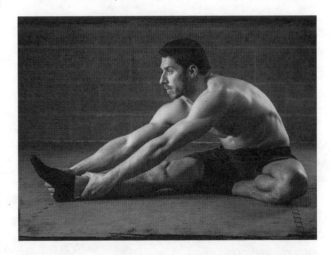

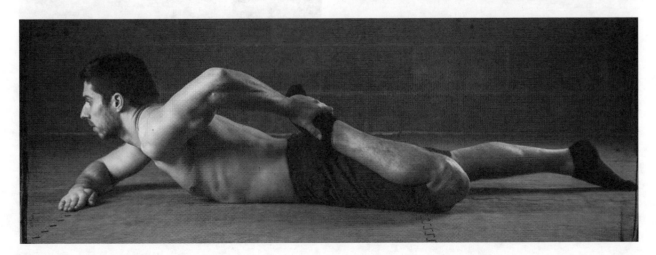

Straddle Stretch

The seated straddle stretch is very good for opening up the hip joint and increasing flexibility of the lower body. Again, this stretch can help with movements and exercises like the planche.

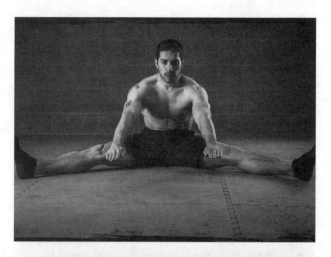

1. Get into a seated position with your legs in the widest "V" position you can manage. Point your toes and fold at the hips, reaching forwards until you feel the stretch.

2. This stretch is also very effective with a partner. Ask them to push on the middle of your back to increase the stretch. Hold for 15 seconds.

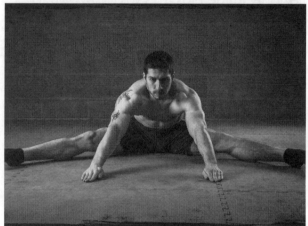

Groin Stretch

The groin, or adductor muscles, allow the hips to be more open and mobile, so to improve flexibility, we can use the seated groin stretch.

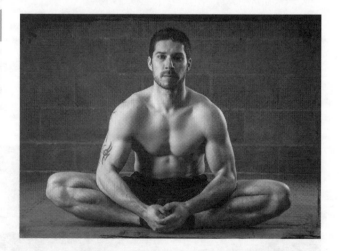

1. Sit down with the soles of your feet together, and pull them in as close to your butt as possible.

2. Sit up straight and attempt to get your knees as low to the floor as possible. You can use the muscles on the outsides of your legs to pull the knees down, or you can simply push on them with your arms or hands. Hold for 15 seconds.

Hip Flexor Stretch

Most people's hip flexors are tight, and this can inhibit the glutes from doing their job. Your jumping and other lower body movements should improve after increasing your hip flexor flexibility.

1. Get into a kneeling position with one leg in front of you. Keep your torso upright and lean forwards.

2. You should feel a stretch in the top of your rear leg. If you don't, then simply increase the distance between the foot and your knee. Hold this position for 15 seconds, change sides and repeat.

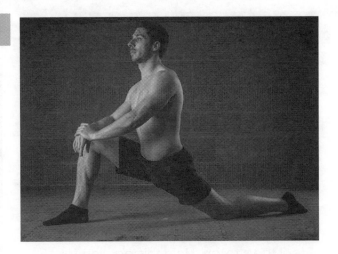

Glute Stretch

The glutes, or butt muscles, are the largest and most powerful in the body, so it is important to stretch them to maintain performance in running, jumping, and other lower body movements.

1. Sit down with one leg straight and the other leg tucked up, with the outside of your foot by the knee of the straight leg.

2. Push the bent knee towards your straight leg until you feel the stretch in your glutes. Hold this position for 15 seconds, change sides and repeat.

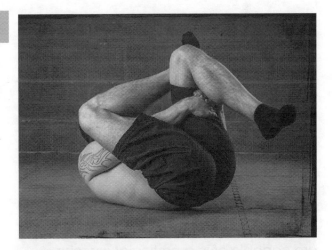

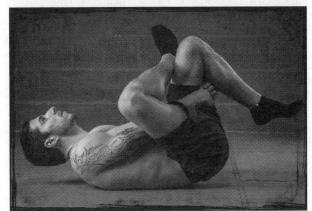

Calf Stretch

The calves, or the bottom of the lower leg, are responsible for pointing the toes and for balance and stability of the foot. If they are tight they can also inhibit the ability of the body to get into a deep squat position.

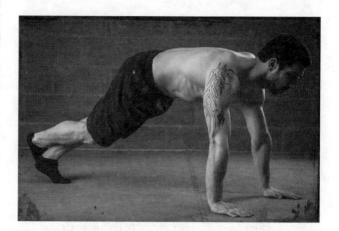

1. Get into a push-up position and place one foot over the other.

2. Now push your heel down until you feel the stretch. Hold this position for 15 seconds, change sides and repeat.

Other Factors

In this section we will look at other factors that relate to the performance of the exercises before looking at the exercises themselves. These factors are: range of motion, using momentum, and cheating on the exercises.

Range of Motion

Range of motion (ROM) refers to the maximum amount of movement your joints are capable of in a particular exercise. For example, if we use the push-up as an example, the maximum range of motion with the hands on the floor would involve starting with the arms locked out, and then lowering down until your chest touches the floor. A reduced range of motion would involve only bending the elbows a small amount, say until they reached 90 degrees.

Range of motion is important because:

• The bigger the range of motion the more difficult the exercise will be, which in turn will make you stronger. This is the case for every exercise that involves the movement of joints. Obviously, mobility and flexibility will also determine how much range of motion you can achieve for certain exercises but, as with all training, time and perseverance will improve both of these qualities.

• It allows you to perform the exercises properly. If we take the pull-up as an example, the most difficult part of the movement is going from a dead hang (where the arms are completely straight) to actually getting the elbows to bend in the pull. If you perform pull-ups and never lower yourself down until your arms are straight, then that part of the movement will always be weak, no matter how much you train the rest of the movement.

Sometimes it is not possible to perform an exercise with complete range of motion, because you might not be strong enough to complete the movement. For example, when you are learning the triceps dip, you may not be strong enough to push yourself up from the bottom position. In these instances it is perfectly fine to work with a reduced ROM until you are strong enough to perform the movement properly.

Using Momentum

Momentum refers to the movement generated by certain exercises that can be used to make the exercise easier. An example of this would be the hanging leg raise. This exercise requires you to hang from a bar and use your core muscles to raise your legs as high as possible before lowering them again. Naturally, when you return the legs to the bottom position, there is the opportunity to use the momentum generated from this action to help with the next repetition. You should strive as much as possible to *not* do this, as using momentum will negate the recruitment of the muscles you are trying to work. In the case of the hanging leg raise, simply ensure that your lower body is stationary before attempting the next repetition.

For the other movements, you will have to be aware of what your body is doing at all times, and if you suspect yourself of using momentum, then slow down and try and perform the exercise with greater discipline. Filming your performance can help as the camera never lies. You can use this method to check your progress, and it also helps to reinforce how much stronger you may be getting over the weeks and months.

"Cheating" at the Exercises

Using momentum isn't the only way that we can "cheat" at an exercise: contorting the body and not keeping rigid form is another way of making the more challenging movements easier. For example, if we take the pull-up again, it is possible to make this exercise much less demanding by raising the legs or knees up to the torso, which shortens the core muscles and makes the pulling action easier. Whilst this is needed sometimes, as in the case of one-arm pull-ups, you should try and stop the practice as soon as possible.

When you are performing the exercises in Part IV, try and maintain your form as perfect as possible at all times, even at the expense of performing fewer repetitions, or using a smaller range of motion. There will be plenty of time to increase the number of repetitions, but the most important point to remember when starting calisthenics is to try and perform each exercise perfectly first. Again, we need to be able to walk before we try to run.

IV The Exercises

Now that you have a little background information and you know how to warm up and prepare your body for the workout, we are going to start looking at the actual calisthenic exercises and the techniques and progressions we can use to work our way to the more advanced movements. I have broken the exercises down into a number of chapters.

Chapter 5: Push-ups

This chapter contains the push-up exercises, including the push-up, clap push-up, pseudo planche push-up, and many others. These movements are all pushing movements in that the hands are moving away from the centre of the body whilst force is being generated. The muscles involved in push-ups include the triceps, forearms, chest, shoulders, and core.

Chapter 6: Pull-ups

This chapter contains the pull-ups and their variations. Included in this section are the pull-up, rock climber, one-arm chin-up, and many others. The pull-up exercises are obviously in the pulling group of movements, so they use the forearms, biceps, back, and core muscle groups.

Chapter 7: Dips

This chapter contains the dip exercises, including, ledge dips, triceps dips, and others. The dip is another pushing exercise, and as such uses the forearms, triceps, shoulders and chest muscle groups.

Chapter 8: Muscle-ups

This chapter contains the muscle-up group of exercises. The muscle-up is a combination of the pull-up and the dip but is much more difficult than either of them to execute, and is unique in that simply being able to perform a pull-up and a dip is not enough to be able to successfully perform a muscle-up.

Chapter 9: Handstands

This chapter contains the handstand exercises, starting with shoulder strengthening and progressing onto free balancing handstands and finally handstand push-ups. Again, these movements are classed as pushing movements but have the added demand of controlling the lower body as well, so that the muscles used are the forearms, shoulders, chest, back, and the core.

Chapter 10: Levers

This chapter contains the lever-based exercises, including, the half lever, front lever, back lever, human flag, and the planche. All these exercises have features in common with each other, which are; strength exerted with straight arms, torso and legs held straight with the joints locked out, and maximum muscular tension throughout the entire body. The levers are the maximal strength exercises in this book, and therefore should only be attempted when a solid foundation has been built.

Chapter 11: Floor Core Exercises

This chapter contains the floor-based core exercises (so require little or no equipment), such as the plank, arch, side plank, dish, dragon flag, plus many others. The muscles used are generally those found in the core. You will find no real isolation exercises in this book, and if your target is a six-pack or to get ripped, then you would do well to read the nutrition section again.

Chapter 12: Leg Raise Exercises

This chapter contains the leg raise exercises, including the knee raise, the leg raise, and the window wiper. All of these are core exercises but they also make some demand on the upper body. They are all performed on a pull-up bar.

Chapter 13: Lower Body Exercises

This chapter contains all of the lower body exercises. The lower body includes movements that use the muscles of the butt, legs, and calves, such as the squat, lunge, and hamstring curl. In athletic movements, the lower body, and especially the hips, are responsible for power production. Sprinting, jumping, running and changing direction, etc., all rely on huge power and strength that originates in the muscles of the glutes, quadriceps, hamstrings, and calves.

Chapter 14: Conditioning Exercises

The conditioning group of exercises is not specifically for strength, but deals with an element that is missing from many peoples' training, known as conditioning. Conditioning exercises make your heart and lungs stronger, and improve the ability of your body to keep going when fatigued. Included in this group of exercises are jumping jacks, burpees, sprints, and many others. You will find that most, if not all, of the exercises in this section use all muscle groups to some extent. For example, the burpee involves pushing, core, and lower body, and in the more advanced variations, such as bastards, all movement possibilities are utilised. Included in this section are the mountain climber, squat thrust, bear crawl, and many other excellent conditioning movements.

The reason that I have broken the exercises down into these particular groups is because calisthenics is not about training individual muscle groups; it is about training movements and whole areas of the body. There is plenty of research on this subject and all agree on one key point; doing multi-joint, multidirectional exercise is far superior to any isolation exercise, especially if you are training for strength, power, and all-round athletic ability.

Before attempting any of the more challenging variations however, it is important to realise that a solid foundation of strength must be built first. This foundation is the key to making good progress using calisthenics, as perfecting the simpler movements will make the more difficult ones easier to tackle. The exercises used in building a solid foundation will probably be well known to you. The push-up, pull-up, triceps dip, squat, and many others are some of the most popular exercises used when anyone begins to train using bodyweight exercises. The difference lies in performing them properly, with perfect technique. Let us take push-ups as an example. Most of the time when I see them being performed, a number of faults occur:

- **The range of motion is nowhere near adequate, with the arms not locking out at the top of the movement and the chest not touching the ground when in the bottom position. Range of movement is very important for proper strength development, and we will talk more about this later.**

- **Poor core stabilisation – this is most often shown by a dipping of the hips when the body is lowered, and also by an arch in the lower back; both are indicative of poor abdominal strength.**

- **The head tilting or jutting forwards – this is indicated by the neck straining forwards and the muscles needed for the proper execution of the push-up not being used. This normally happens because the person in question tries to progress too fast. This also reduces the range of motion, as the head will get close to the ground before the chest and torso does.**

All of these issues and more add up to many people not being able to perform even a simple exercise like the push-up perfectly, even if they are convinced that they can. In my experience this is only because the person in question will have moved on from simple bodyweight exercises before they are ready, or because they do not appreciate the amount of time it takes to build real, useable strength. It goes without saying that if you cannot perform the simpler version(s) of an exercise, you should not progress onto the more difficult version(s). You may think that you are performing it properly, but the chances are that you will be fooling yourself, and even if your progress is quick to begin with, it will soon slow when attempting some of the more challenging exercises.

Another reason why starting simple and slow is best when it comes to calisthenics is that many of the movements are extremely taxing on the body. Many people do not realise this because exercises just using the bodyweight are traditionally seen as easier than ones that use dumbbells and barbells. This is simply not the case. Most, if not all, of the weighted exercises can be learnt and performed properly in a relatively short amount of time. Once the bench press is learnt, then you gradually add more weight and increase the resistance. Once the deadlift is learnt, then more weight is added to the bar and progress is made. However, if we take an exercise such as the front lever, it is impossible for someone to just learn the movement and be expected to perform it the same way as a dumbbell or barbell exercise. To get to the stage where a solid front lever can be performed takes months and months of slow steady progression, where all of the variations of the exercise have to be perfected before moving on to the next progression. A similar phenomenon is seen with the one-arm pull-up. Not only is the one-arm pull-up extremely taxing on the muscles, it also puts a huge strain on the ligaments and tendons. It is simply not possible for the majority of people to jump in to performing the high-level exercises with no prior experience.

As such, in the following chapters, there are some exercises that are very important to master before you move on to the more advanced ones. These **Fundamental Five**, as I have called them, and the number of sets and repetitions that you must work up to, are as follows:

- **Push-ups – minimum of 20 perfect repetitions**

- **Pull-ups – minimum of 10 perfect repetitions**

- **Triceps dips – minimum of 10 perfect repetitions**

- **Hanging knee raises – minimum of 10 perfect repetitions**

- **Squats – minimum of 25 perfect repetitions**

Now that we have learnt exactly what exercises are included, and why, it is time to start working on them. Within each exercise there are three sections:

1. **An explanation of the exercise and any important information.**

2. **The description of the exercise itself with pictures of each stage.**

3. **A teaching points section, which will help you with any problems that you may have.**

The push-up is perhaps the best known bodyweight exercise, and even if you are not a regular exerciser you will have probably done a few of them, either at school or at some point in your life. They are used perhaps most commonly in militaries around the world, as it is easy to teach, very effective, and requires no specialist equipment.

In its simplest form, the push-up requires you to push your body away from the floor, supporting yourself on your toes and keeping your core tight. The more advanced variations, such as the handstand push-up and planche push-up, require extreme levels of strength, even though you will only be using your bodyweight. In gymnastics, the push-up is used to develop wrist strength, shoulder stability, pushing power, and core strength. It is also useful as an exercise in a circuit.

In this chapter we will start by looking at the standard push-up, and take time to ensure that we can perform it perfectly before moving on. In many cases people I have trained are too eager to move to the more advanced exercises, but do not underestimate the benefits of doing simple movements extremely well.

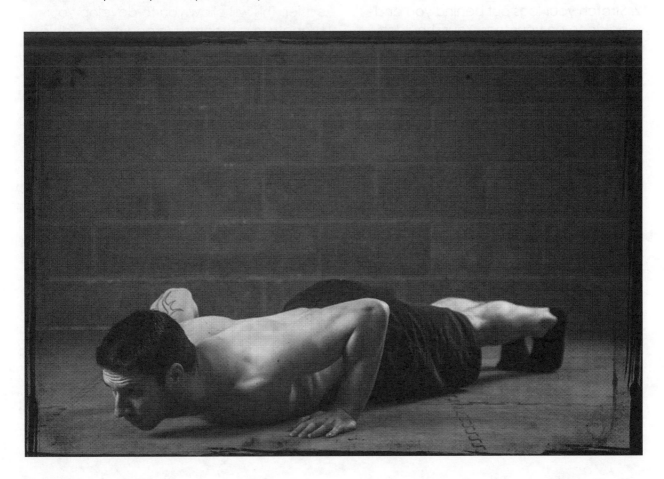

Push-up

As was mentioned in the introduction to this chapter, the push-up is the most well-known bodyweight exercise and the starting point for the exercise part of this book: do not be tempted to move on until you can perform it perfectly. It may not seem like it, but how well you can perform a push-up determines to a large degree how well you will progress with other movements. It tests your upper body strength and control, your ability to keep the core tight, and the ability to generate muscular tension throughout the body as a whole.

1. Place your hands on the floor shoulder width apart.

2. Stretch your legs out behind you and balance on your toes. Your shoulders, hips, knees, and feet should form a straight line.

3. Keeping your eyes looking forwards at about 45 degrees, bend your elbows and start to lower yourself down to the ground.

4. Allow your elbows to push out slightly from the torso, and stop when your chest touches the ground. At this point only your chest and toes should be touching the floor.

5. Pause for a split second, and then push down hard, straightening your arms until you reach the start position. This counts as one repetition. You should be aiming to perform 3 sets of 10 repetitions.

Teaching Points

If you do not have enough strength to perform the push-up, it needs to be made easier. This will allow you to develop your strength in a progressive and measurable manner. The simplest and best way to increase pushing strength for the push-up is to use a raised platform for the hands to rest on. This alters the angle of the body and moves more or less weight from the hands to the feet. The rule for this method is that if the hands are higher than the feet then the movement will be easier, and if the feet are raised higher than the hands then the exercise will be more difficult. Work with the hands raised and as you become stronger, simply reduce the height of the platform until you can perform the push-up with your hands on the floor.

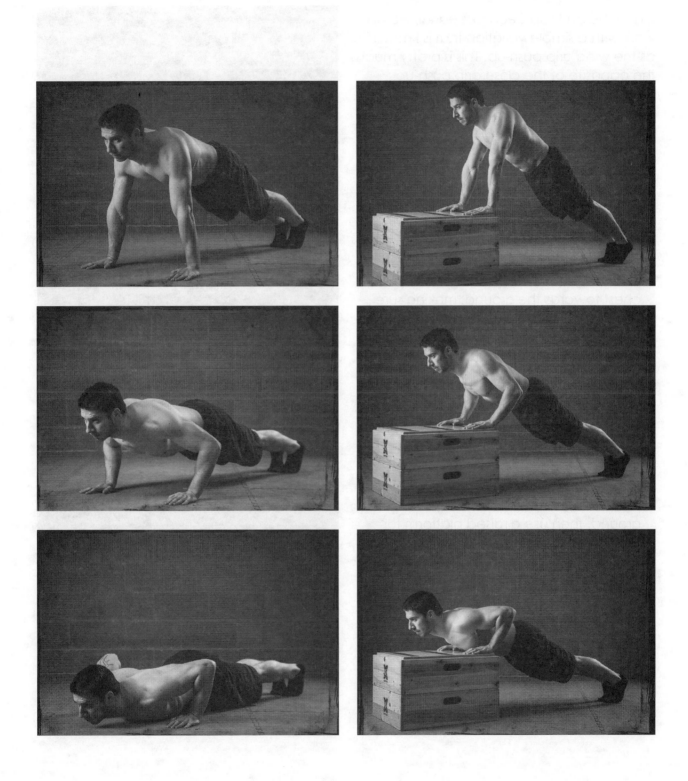

Wide Grip Push-up

Once the push-up becomes easier, we can work with a simple variation that is known as the wide grip push-up. This is pretty much the opposite of the close grip push-up (see opposite page), in that the hands are placed on the floor in as wide a position as possible. This version uses the muscles of the chest much more than in the standard or close grip push-up.

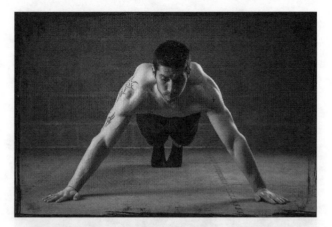

1. Get into the push-up position. From here, move your hands as wide apart as you can.

2. Now bend your elbows and lower your chest towards the ground, making sure to keep your shoulders, hips, knees and toes in a straight line. As your hands are placed wider apart you can allow your elbows to shoot out to the sides.

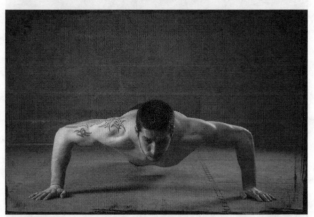

3. Keep going down until your chest touches the ground, then push back up as hard as you can until you reach the start position. This counts as one repetition. Again, if you have trouble performing this with your feet on the ground, then use a raised platform for the hands, as described on page 78. You should again try and perform 3 sets of 10 repetitions.

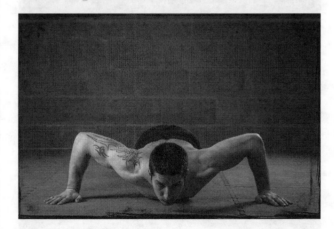

Close Grip Push-up

Another variation of the push-up is the close grip push-up where the hands are closer together. It is an excellent exercise for targeting the triceps muscles as the elbows are kept tight into the sides which makes the movement much more difficult. You are likely to find this variation much harder than the ones presented so far, but this is normal.

1. Get into the push-up position. From here, move your hands closer together until they are touching.

2. Now bend your elbows and lower your chest towards the ground, making sure to keep your shoulders, hips, knees and toes in a straight line. Keep your elbows tucked into your sides. If you can make them brush your ribs, as shown in the pictures, then you will be targeting the correct muscle groups.

3. Keep going down until your chest touches your hands, then push back up as hard as you can until you reach the start position. This counts as one repetition. Again, if you have trouble performing this with your feet on the ground, then use a raised platform for the hands, as described on page 78. You should again try and perform 3 sets of 10 repetitions.

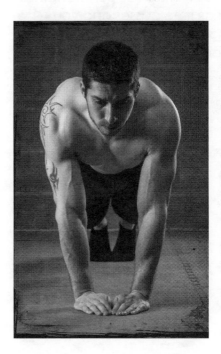
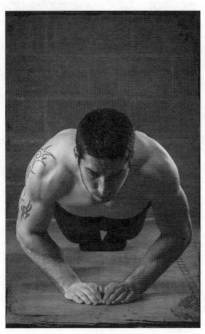
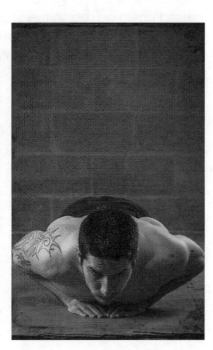

Deep Push-up

Once the push-up becomes a little too easy, or if you want a bit more of a challenge, you can try the deep push-up. This variation is simply where the range of motion is as large as we can make it, whilst still using the same hand grip and body position of the standard push-up. For this, you will need either push-up bars or parallettes, or two objects of equal height that you can place your hands on.

1. Place your hands on the apparatus you are using to elevate your hands, and get into the push-up position.

2. From here, bend your elbows and lower yourself down as far as possible. You should aim to get your chest well below the level of your hands to achieve as much range of motion as possible.

3. When you are down as deep as your flexibility and strength allow, push up hard until you reach the start position. This counts as one repetition. Again, you should try and perform 3 sets of 10 repetitions.

Teaching Points

When starting out with deep push-ups you may struggle to get any real depth at all. This will increase with time though, as will the flexibility of the shoulders. To begin with, only lower yourself as far as your strength will allow, and as time passes and you become stronger, try and increase the range of motion as much as physically possible.

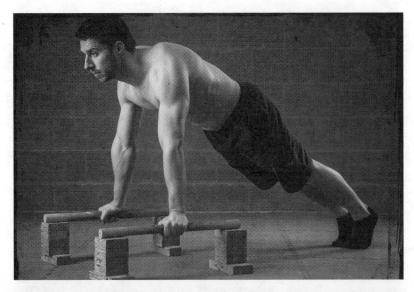

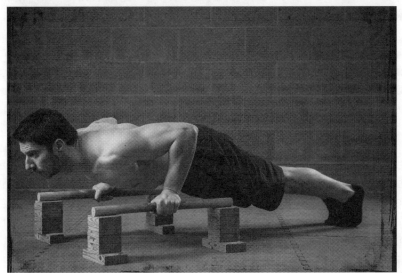

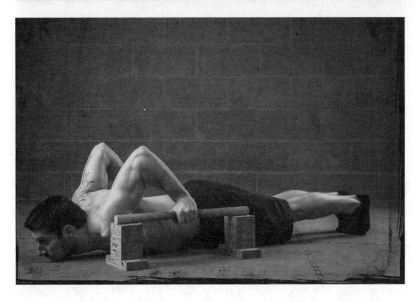

Archer Push-up

The archer push-up is another unusual push-up variation, and introduces the concept of straight-arm strength that we looked at in the introduction. If you are competent with the one-arm push-up (see page 94), then you should not have too much trouble with the archer push-up. It is extremely important in this exercise that you keep the elbow **completely locked**. With straight-arm exercises, even a slightly bent elbow will make the movement easier and in effect defeats the object of keeping the arm straight.

1. Get into the wide grip push-up position.

2. From here, bend one elbow of one arm but keep the other absolutely straight. Move your bodyweight over the bent arm as you lower yourself down.

3. As you do this, keep the straight arm locked at the elbow, and keep going until your chest touches the ground. It can help here to look towards the straight arm to ensure that your technique and form is correct, as you can see in the pictures.

4. From here, push up with your bent arm and try and pull through the floor with the straight one, until you reach the start position. This counts as one repetition.

Teaching Points

Working with archer push-ups if you are not familiar with straight-arm work can be daunting at first. The main problem is that of not having the ability to keep the arm completely locked as you move through the exercise, and this is actually easier said than done. The body will want to bend the elbow, mainly to protect the joint, as a locked joint is a weaker one, especially when we are trying to exert some strength and power. To counteract this, it is important to make sure that your form remains perfect and be very vigilant on how straight your arm is at all times.

In terms of sets and repetitions, you should aim to perform 3 sets of 5 repetitions on each arm, alternating on each repetition.

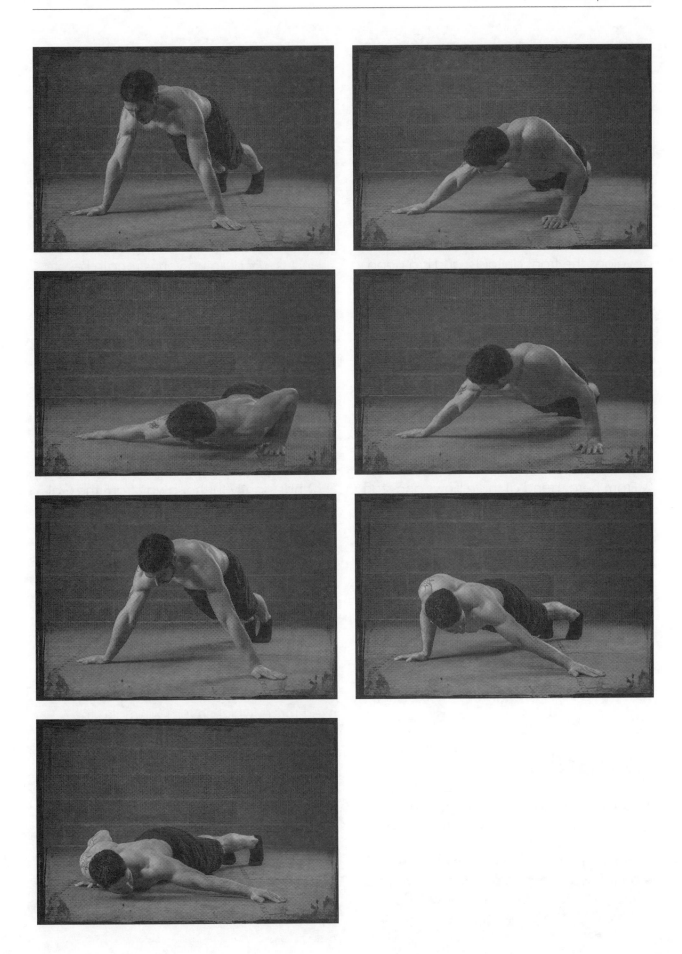

Wall Push-up

The wall push-up is another push-up exercise that makes heavy use of the core. It involves placing the feet on a sturdy wall and whilst the body is horizontal, performing a push-up. It is much more difficult than it sounds, mainly because it requires the shoulders to push the feet into the wall hard, so that they do not slip down the wall. This exercise also really develops the front deltoids, and is a good preparation exercise for the planche, which is covered in Chapter 10.

1. Face away from a wall and place your feet at the bottom of it. Keeping your arms locked, walk your feet onto the wall until they reach the same height as your shoulders. Ensure that you keep this strict position throughout the whole movement.

2. From here, bend at the elbows and start to lower your chest towards the ground. At the same time walk your feet down the wall towards the ground in small steps, so that your entire body stays as horizontal as possible.

3. Once your chest touches the ground, push back up until your arms are straight. At the same time walk your feet back up the wall until you reach the start position. This counts as one repetition.

Teaching Points

When first starting with the wall push-up, you are likely to run into two problems.

1. The first is that when you hold yourself on the wall, your core droops down and you get a large arch in the lower back. This is down to poor core strength and will improve with core training and time. If you cannot hold the straight body position at the same time as walking up and down the wall, then simply hold the start position for as long as you can, and slowly build up your strength before moving onto the push-up variation.

2. The second issue is that of not being able to push back hard enough with the shoulders to keep the feet glued onto the wall. Remember, the only factor keeping your feet on the wall is the friction of your shoes or feet on the surface of the wall, and the ability of your shoulders and arms to push your body against the wall. To make this easier you can move your hands slightly further away from the wall. This will mean that you will be pushing marginally more in an overhead position than before, which should make keeping your feet on the wall slightly easier.

In addition, the method of moving the hands forwards to make the movement easier can be altered and used to make the exercise more challenging. By moving the hands closer to the wall we can decrease the ability of the shoulders to exert force, which in turn will make the exercise more difficult. This is the same principle that is used with the pseudo planche push-up (see page 92), where the hands are moved behind the shoulders to increase the challenge.

When you start this exercise you should aim for 3 sets of 10 repetitions. As you progress and move your hands towards the wall, you will have to reduce the number of repetitions.

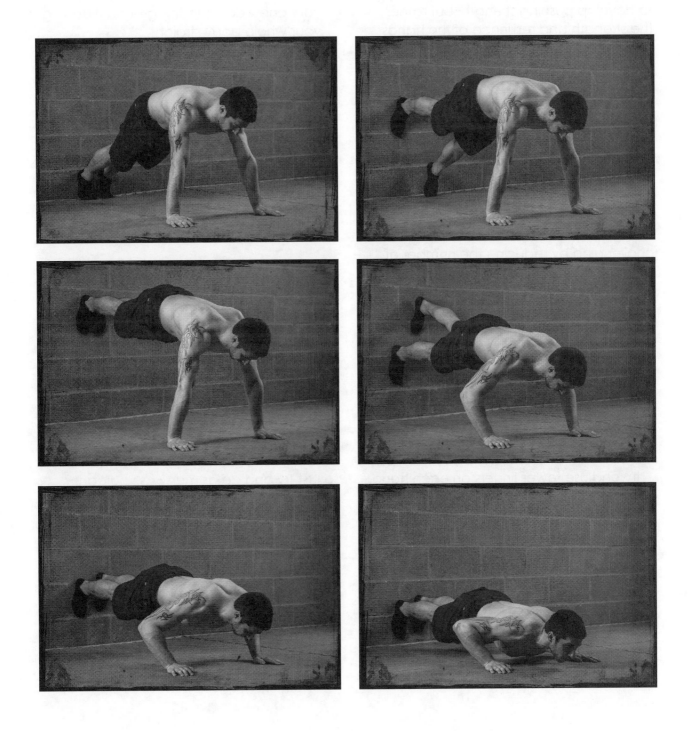

Fingertip Push-up

The fingertip push-up is not necessarily used to develop pushing strength, but rather the strength and resilience of the hands and fingers. Hand strength is an extremely overlooked part of physical training, but without it you cannot hope to reach your full potential. As with the scapulae, training the hands and the fingers is vital in being able to perform some of the more challenging calisthenic exercises. Fingertip push-ups do well to introduce you to the type of hand and finger strength needed to progress. As your hands become stronger, you can make this exercise more challenging by reducing the number of fingers that you use on each hand.

1. Get into the push-up position, but instead of supporting yourself on your palms, raise yourself up onto your fingertips. It helps to try and spread the fingers out and place most of the stress through the thumb joint, as this is much stronger than the other joints of the hand. As you can see, I am using all of the five fingers and thumbs on each hand. As you progress, try and use fewer fingers on each hand.

2. From here, bend at the elbows and lower your chest down to the ground, keeping your whole body straight.

3. Once your chest reaches the ground, push up hard until you reach the start position. This counts as one repetition.

Teaching Points

For this exercise you should try and perform 3 sets of 10 repetitions. Depending upon the strength in your hands, you may feel more stress in your fingers than you do in your upper body so you may have to stop before you reach 10 repetitions. This is fine, so just try and do as many as you can.

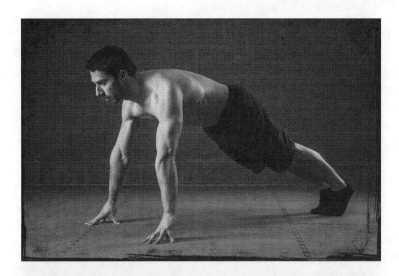

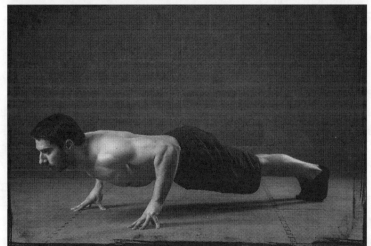

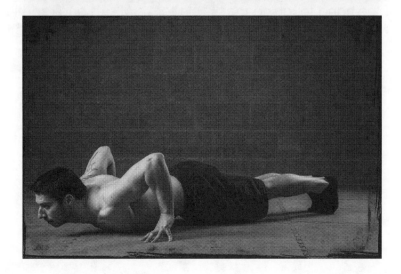

Wrist Push-up

Like the fingertip push-up, the wrist push-up is another very good exercise that can be used to strengthen an area that is very important in other areas of calisthenics. The wrists are another weak link in the upper body chain, and it does not matter how strong the rest of your upper body is, if the wrists are weak, it will fail there. Remember the old saying, 'a chain is only as strong as its weakest link'.

Wrist push-ups are very difficult for most people, especially if they have never performed any wrist strengthening exercises before. Ensure that you take your time with them and do not push yourself too hard too soon.

1. Place your knees on the ground and position the backs of your hands on the ground with your fingers pointing inwards.

2. From here, bend your elbows and lower your chest down towards the floor. It helps here to try and keep the hand as flat as possible at all times, as this will ensure that you have the biggest possible area of the hand touching the ground, which will aid in stability and comfort.

3. From this bottom position, push-up hard until your arms become straight again. This counts as one repetition.

Teaching Points

For some people, even performing wrist push-ups on the knees is too difficult. To remedy this, simply use the method that we looked at for the push-up, i.e. using a raised platform or box to place the hands on. As before, the higher the hands in relation to the feet, or in this case the knees, the easier the movement will become. Once performing the movement on your knees becomes too easy, you can raise yourself up onto your toes and perform the exercise in the same way as a push-up.

In terms of sets and repetitions, start by aiming for 3 sets of 5 repetitions, and then build up from there.

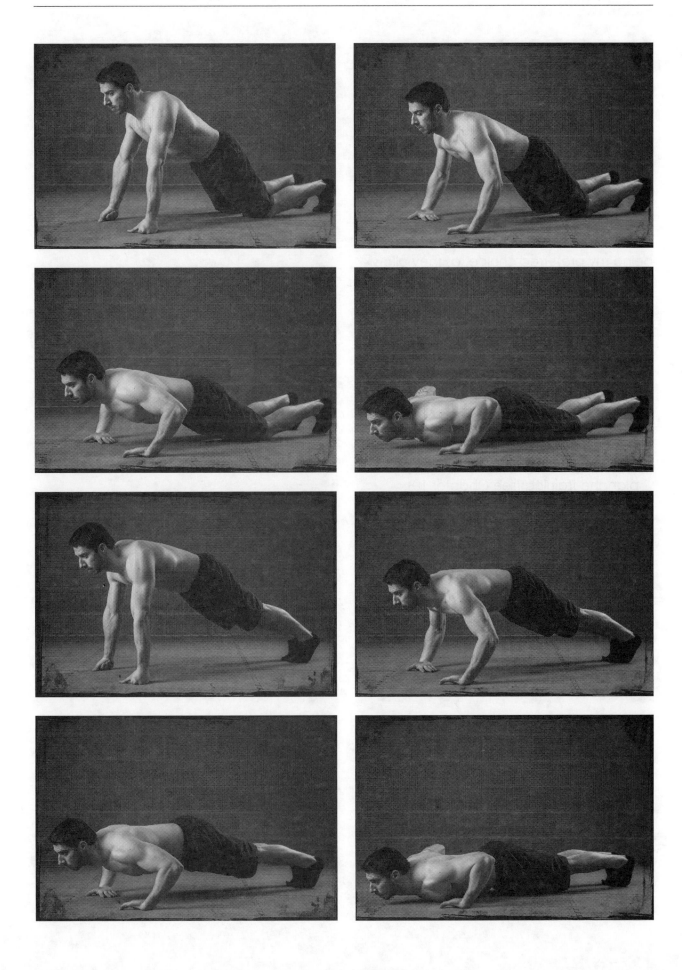

Pseudo Planche Push-up

The pseudo planche press-up is an extremely deceptive exercise, as it looks almost identical to a press-up except that the shoulders are moved further forwards than the hands. It is this that makes it so challenging. This movement also gives you a taste of what it feels like to train the planche. You can either use the floor or parallettes for this exercise, with parallettes being my preferred choice, as they allow a greater degree of control than just using the floor.

1. Get into the push-up position. You can turn your hands out slightly here to help with any flexibility issues. Walk forwards on your toes until your shoulders are further forwards than your hands. Try and keep your elbows straight at this stage, as this will strengthen the biceps and the tendons of the elbow in preparation for planche training (see Chapter 10).

2. Now bend you elbows and lower your chest to the floor, making sure to keep your shoulders in front of your hands at all times.

3. Once your chest reaches the floor, push back up to the start position, ensuring that your arms lock out at the top of the movement. This counts as one repetition. Try and perform 3 sets of 6 repetitions.

Teaching Points

For most people, the ability to hold the body in an unnatural position (that of the shoulders in front of the hands) is very difficult. To begin with, try only moving forwards of the hands a small amount, increasing the distance between the hands and the shoulders as you become stronger.

The ultimate aim of this exercise is to end up with your hands as close to your hips as possible at the bottom of the movement. You will have to be strict with yourself when performing this exercise, as it is quite easy to cheat. Try watching your form in a mirror, video it, or ask a training partner to help you.

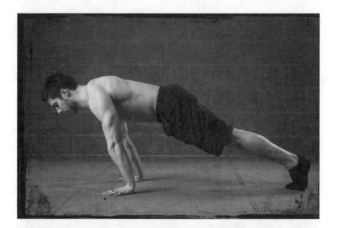

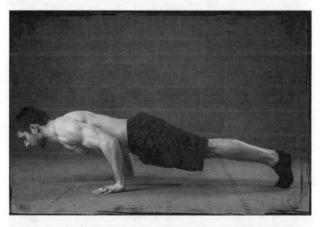

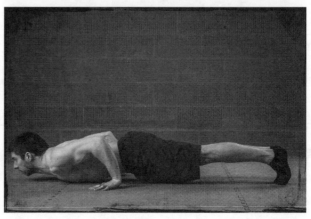

Lalanne Push-up

The Lalanne push-up is named after the famous "Godfather of Fitness" Jack Lalanne, who was an American fitness, exercise, and nutritional expert. Jack lived in California and did untold amounts towards promoting healthy living during his lifetime. A holder of numerous world records, he was often seen performing this movement.

The Lalanne push-up is as much a test of core strength as it is of pushing strength. It is identical in its starting position to the extended plank, and will give you a good idea of exerting core strength when the core musculature is stretched out. It is a little less of a push-up than the ones we have looked at so far, as the arms will not really do that much pushing. You can think of this movement as a kind of bridge, where we are trying to span a very wide river. It goes without saying that the wider the river, the stronger the bridge has to be, and this is why this movement is so effective at building strength.

1. Get into the push-up position.

2. From here, walk your hands forwards until you are as stretched out as you can manage.

3. Now lower yourself down until your body touches the ground. Ensure to keep plenty of tension in the body and the torso.

4. From this bottom position, push with your upper body and contract your core muscles as strongly as possible until you reach the start position. As you can see my arms are not bending that much, and it is really my core that is acting to raise the body off the ground. This counts as one repetition.

Teaching Points

When first starting the Lalanne push-up it may not be possible for you to stretch out as far as is shown in the pictures. To make it more manageable, simply move the hands a little closer to the feet. This will shorten the core and put the core musculature into a stronger position, making the exercise easier. As you become stronger, simply start to move the hands and feet further apart until you are fully stretched out.

In terms of sets and repetitions, you should begin by trying to do 3 sets of 5 repetitions and build from there. You will probably find that your core becomes tired before your upper body, but as this is a core exercise as well, this is not a problem.

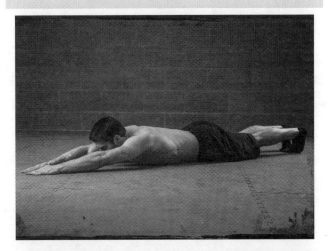

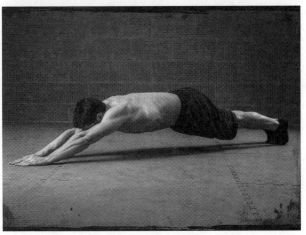

One-Arm Push-up

The one-arm push-up has achieved almost cult status amongst the fitness crowd, but nonetheless it is still an extremely useful exercise, not just for the upper body, but also for the core. There is a fair amount of technique involved, and quite a lot of balance, but it can be achieved by anyone with enough hard work and perseverance. One reason that it is very effective and useful for us as calisthenic practitioners is that it is a unilateral exercise, which simply means that it uses only one limb, or only one side of the body. Another example would be the single-leg squat, or the one-arm chin-up. These movements are rightly considered some of the most challenging bodyweight exercises, and really help to develop some of the extreme strength that we are trying to build.

1. Place one hand on the floor and position your chest over the top of your hand. Place your feet wider apart than normal to aid in your balance. Place your free arm behind your back or by your side.

2. Now bend your elbow and lower yourself down as far as you can, whilst keeping your body straight. You will no doubt have to lean over to one side to keep your balance, but this is perfectly normal and is allowed.

3. As soon as you are as low as possible, push up hard from the floor until you reach the start position. This counts as one repetition. You should aim to perform 3 sets of 3 to 5 repetitions on each arm.

Teaching Points

There are two main methods to build up your strength for the one-arm push-up.

1. The first method is to perform the movement on a raised platform, as described in the push-up (see page 78). Again, the higher the platform you use, the easier the movement will be. As you become stronger you can simply reduce the height of the box or platform you are using until you can perform the movement on the floor.

2. The second method is where we use the free arm to assist with the movement. Use a raised platform for your free hand to do this. To start with, position yourself close to the platform and get into the one-arm push-up stance. Place your free hand on the platform and attempt to perform a one-arm push-up. If you need to, use your free hand to help push up. As you become stronger, simply increase the distance between you and the platform. This has the effect of reducing the amount of help that your free arm can offer. Keep moving the platform further and further away until you are using only your fingertips with a straight arm to help push back up. Once you have achieved this, it will only be a short time until you are able to perform the movement on the floor with no assistance.

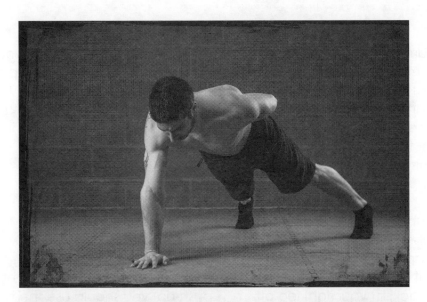

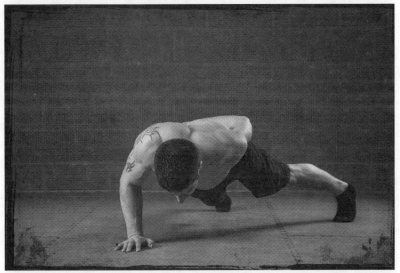

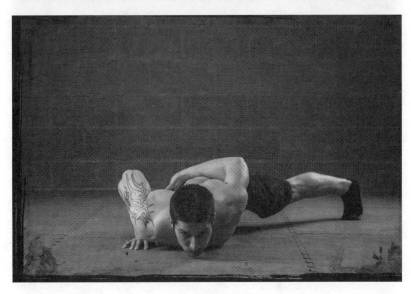

One-Arm One-Leg Push-up

Once the one-arm push-up starts to become a little more straightforward, you can attempt the next stage, which is to raise one leg into the air and perform the one-arm, one-leg variation. Most people discover that whilst their strength is adequate for this movement, their balance lets them down.

1. Get into a push-up position. Raise one arm, place it behind your back, and then lift the opposite leg off the floor. For example, if you place your left arm behind your back, lift your right leg off the ground, and vice versa.

2. Keeping your torso as straight as possible, start to bend your arm and lower your chest to the ground.

3. Once you have lowered yourself as low as you are able to, push up hard until you return to the start position. This counts as one repetition. You should aim to perform 3 sets of 3 to 5 repetitions on each arm.

Teaching Points

To progress with the one-arm one-leg push-up, you should use the two methods outlined for the one-arm push-up, which was using a raised platform and using the free arm to assist with the exercise. Keep progressing until you can perform the movement on the floor with no assistance.

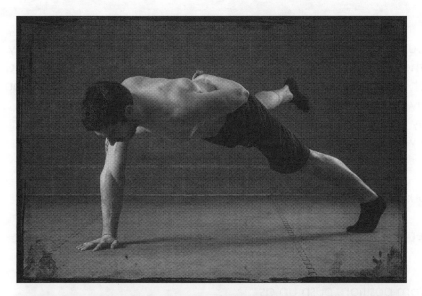

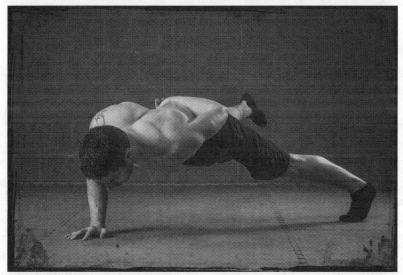

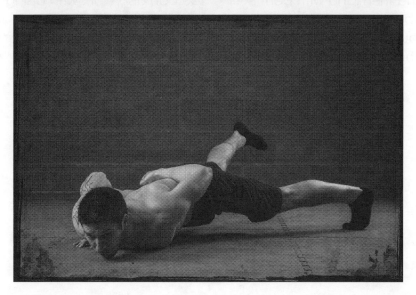

Superman Push-up

The superman push-up, just like the clap push-up, is another example of a group of movements that are known as plyometric. Plyometric simply means powerful, and more specifically when either one part of the body or the whole body leaves the ground.

1. Assume the push-up position.

2. From here, bend your elbows and lower your chest down towards the floor.

3. From this bottom position, push up as hard and as powerfully as you can.

4. As soon as your arms are nearly straight, shove off the ground hard and raise your hands into the air.

5. Once you are in the air try and stretch your arms out into a superman position. The aim is to get them completely straight out in front of your head, so that your body resembles superman in flight.

6. Once you reach full extension, bring your hands back into your torso as fast as you can, and then land with bent elbows. Absorb the shock of the landing by lowering your chest down towards the ground, and then continue with the next repetition.

As this is a power exercise, try and perform 3 sets of 3 to 5 repetitions and then increase the number that you perform as you become stronger.

Teaching Points

Do not worry if you cannot stretch your arms out to the full superman position to begin with. Simply move them out as far as your strength and confidence will allow, and then as you become more powerful and more familiar with the exercise, you will be able to extend further and further.

You can also work with a single arm variation, which will give you the confidence to progress onto the full superman push-up. This is shown in the pictures opposite.

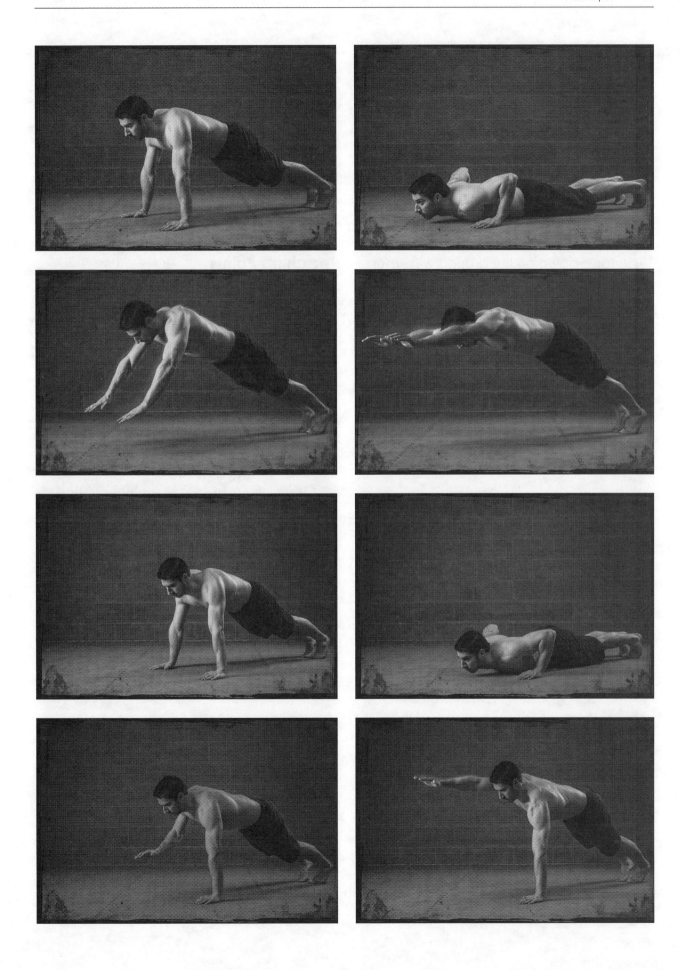

Spider Push-up

The spider push-up is one of the last push-up variations that we will look at and also one of the most difficult. It is similar in principle to the Lalanne push-up (see page 93), in that the hands are held far away from the body, which decreases the leverage and therefore makes the movement much more challenging.

1. Lie face down on the ground with your arms stretched out to the sides. Position your fingertips on the floor.

2. From here, push down hard on the ground with your hands and lift your chest off the floor. Due to the way your body is positioned, you will not be able to rise off the ground a huge amount.

3. Keep pushing until your elbows are locked and your body is held rigid.

4. Now lower yourself back down to the start position. This counts as one repetition.

Teaching Points

At first it may be too challenging to raise yourself off the ground when your arms are fully extended, so begin by positioning your hands closer to your body. This will allow you to exert more strength initially, and then as you become stronger, simply move your hands further and further away from the body.

As the leverage is very decreased in this exercise, it may not be possible for you to perform many repetitions of the movement in one go. Try 3 sets of 5 repetitions initially, and then build up from there.

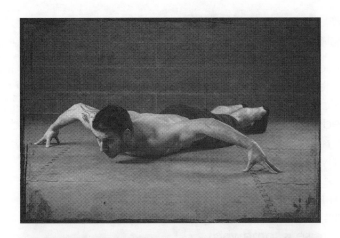

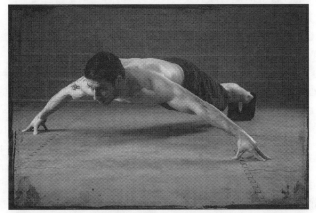

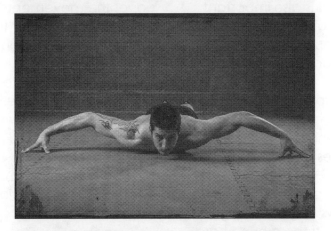

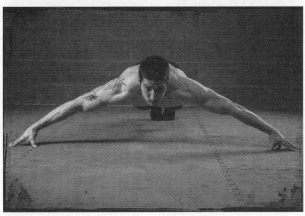

Clap Push-up

A very good variation on the push-up is the clap push-up, sometimes called the explosive or plyometric push-up. Plyometric is simply the word used to signify power usage in an exercise, normally associated with a part of the body leaving the ground, as in a jump or bound. For this exercise the feet will be staying on the ground but the hands will be leaving it to perform a single clap in midair. This exercise is somewhat more dangerous than the others that we have looked at so far, as there is the risk of hurting the hands or of landing on the chest or face if you do not place your hands back into position in time. As always with the more advanced exercises, take your time and only progress when you feel ready.

Ideally, you should protect your hands by using a mat of some kind to absorb the shock of the landing. It is also important that your feet are on a non-slip surface, because you want your feet to remain planted whilst your hands are in the air.

1. Get into the push-up position.

2. Bend you elbows and lower yourself down until your chest touches the floor.

3. From here, push up as powerfully as you can. As your elbows begin to straighten, really try and push off the ground hard, aiming to get your entire upper body to rise into the air.

4. As soon as your hands leave the ground, bring them together in front of your chest and clap quickly, before moving them back to their initial position. Spot the ground and try to "catch" the floor, making an attempt to bend the elbows as soon as you land and descend into the next repetition. This counts as one repetition.

Teaching Points

If you do not have the strength to push up hard enough, practice the push-up, but really concentrate on pushing as hard and as powerfully as possible. We can also use the raised platform method we have looked at a number of times previously. As before, the higher the platform you use, the easier the movement will be, and simply reduce the height of the box as you build strength and confidence.

It is vitally important to lower yourself down until your chest is level with the hands. If you don't, you simply will not have the power or leverage to push your hands off the floor. To gain the strength necessary for this movement, it is important to perform all of the push-up variations with the biggest range of motion that you can.

As the clap push-up is a power movement, it is not really possible to do as many repetitions as the other push-up variations. As this is the case, aim for 3 sets of 5 to 8 repetitions, trying to push yourself as far as you can.

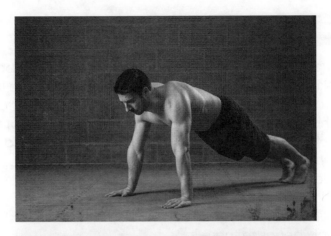

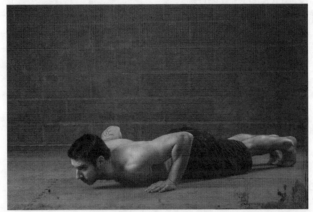

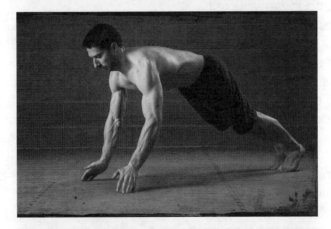

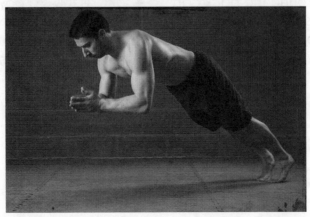

Back Clap Push-up

Once the clap push-up becomes too easy, or if you are looking for an additional challenge, you can start training with the back clap push-up. This, as the name suggests, requires you to clap once behind your back before returning your hands to the front of your body to land again. I should not have to tell you that this is more difficult and considerably more risky than the clap push-up, simply because there is a chance that you will not get your hands back in time to land. For this reason it is best to start with this movement only when you are completely comfortable with the clap push-up. Again, it is advisable for this movement to use some sort of mat to help soften the impact and save the hands and wrists from damage or injury.

1. Get into the push-up position.

2. Bend your elbows and lower yourself down until your chest touches the floor.

3. From here, push up as powerfully as you can. As your elbows start to straighten, really try and shove off the ground hard, aiming to get your entire upper body to rise into the air.

4. As soon as your hands leave the ground, whip them around your torso and clap once behind your back. The action of moving the hands around the back can also give a little boost to your height, so make sure that you really whip them round!

5. Move your hands back in front of your chest ready for the landing. Spot the ground and try to "catch" the floor, making an attempt to bend the elbows as soon as you land and descend into the next repetition. One push-up counts as one repetition.

Teaching Points

As before, the best method for developing back clap push-ups is to use a raised platform for the hands. Start with a high platform and then as you become stronger and more confident, reduce the height of the box until you can perform the exercise on the ground.

Again, as this is a power movement, it will not be possible to do lots of repetitions. Try and perform 3 sets of 3 to 5 repetitions to start with and build from there.

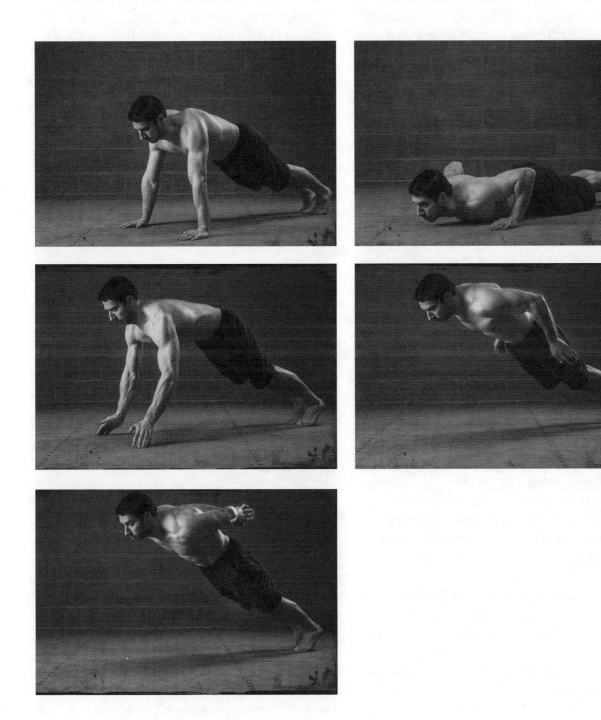

Double Clap Push-up

Once you have more or less mastered both the clap push-up and the back clap push-up, you can attempt to combine them both into a single movement, to create the double clap push-up. As the name suggests, this is where you clap once in front of the body and once behind, before moving the hands back in front of you in time to land. This again is more risky than the back clap push-up, as you have to make sure that you push off hard enough to spend sufficient time in the air to be able to clap twice.

1. Get into the push-up position.

2. Bend your elbows and lower yourself down until your chest touches the floor.

3. From here, push up as powerfully as you can. As your elbows start to straighten, really try and shove off the ground hard, aiming to get your entire upper body to rise into the air.

4. As soon as your hands leave the ground, clap once in front of your chest. It is vital that you perform this clap as quickly as possible, to give you more time to perform the clap behind the back and get the hands back in time to land.

5. Once you have performed the first clap in front of the chest, whip your hands around your torso and clap once behind your back. The action of moving the hands around the back can also give a little boost to your height, so make sure that you really whip them round!

6. Move your hands back in front of your chest ready for the landing. Spot the ground and try to "catch" the floor, making an attempt to bend the elbows as soon as you land and descend into the next repetition. One push-up counts as one repetition.

Teaching Points

As before, the best method for developing double clap push-ups is to use a raised platform for the hands. Start with a high platform and then as you become stronger and more confident, reduce the height of the box until you can perform the exercise on the ground.

As for the number of sets and repetitions, the double clap push-up is extremely taxing, so 3 or 4 sets of 2 to 5 repetitions will be more than enough to begin with.

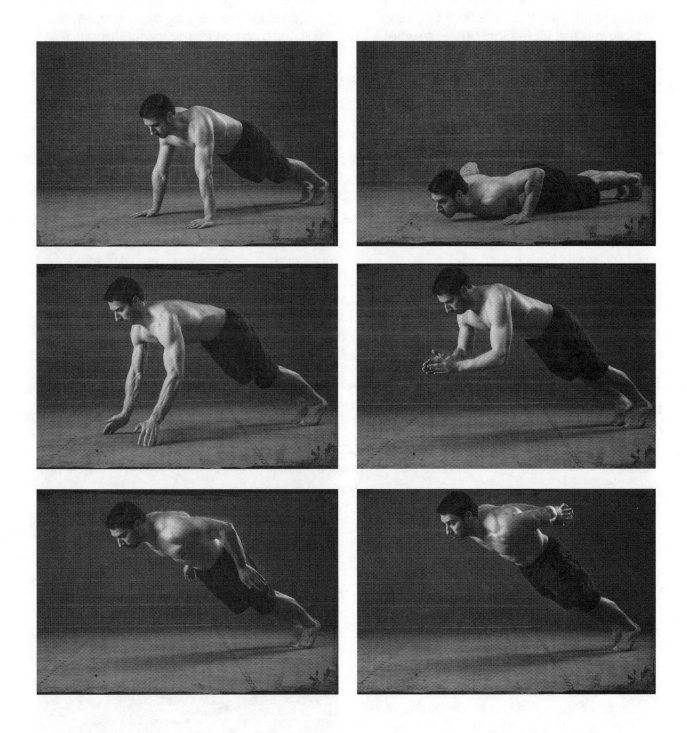

Triple Clap Push-up

If you have achieved the double clap push-up and are still not satisfied with the level of difficulty, then the final clapping variation is the triple clap push-up, where you explode off the ground, clap in front of your body, behind your back, in front of your body, and then land. Even more power is required for this movement, and should only be attempted when you feel that you have enough strength and power to propel yourself high enough into the air to actually complete the movement. Again, a mat or other soft surface is advised, not just in case you land awkwardly, but also to protect the hands and the wrists from the impact.

1. Get into the push-up position.

2. Bend your elbows and lower yourself down until your chest touches the floor.

3. From here, push up as powerfully as you can. As your elbows start to straighten, really try and shove off the ground hard, aiming to get your entire upper body to rise into the air.

4. As soon as your hands leave the ground, clap once in front of your chest. It is vital that you perform this clap as soon as possible, as the quicker you do this the more time you will have to perform the other two claps before you land.

5. Once you have performed the first clap in front of the chest, whip your hands around your torso and clap once behind your back. The action of moving the hands around the back can also give a little boost to your height.

6. Move your hands in front of your chest and clap once more. Again, this action will need to be very quick, because you will need to get ready for the landing afterwards. Spot the ground and try to "catch" the floor, making an attempt to bend the elbows as soon as you land and descend into the next repetition. One push-up counts as one repetition.

Teaching Points

As before, the best method for developing triple clap push-ups is to use a raised platform for the hands. Start with a high platform and then as you become stronger and more confident, reduce the height of the box until you can perform the exercise on the ground.

In terms of sets and repetitions, for this exercise you may only be able to perform a single repetition to begin with. Start with 3 sets of 1 or 2 repetitions, and then build from there when you are ready.

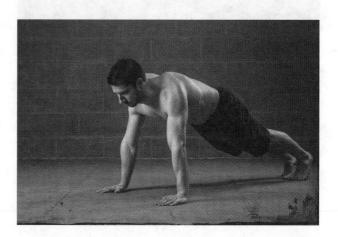

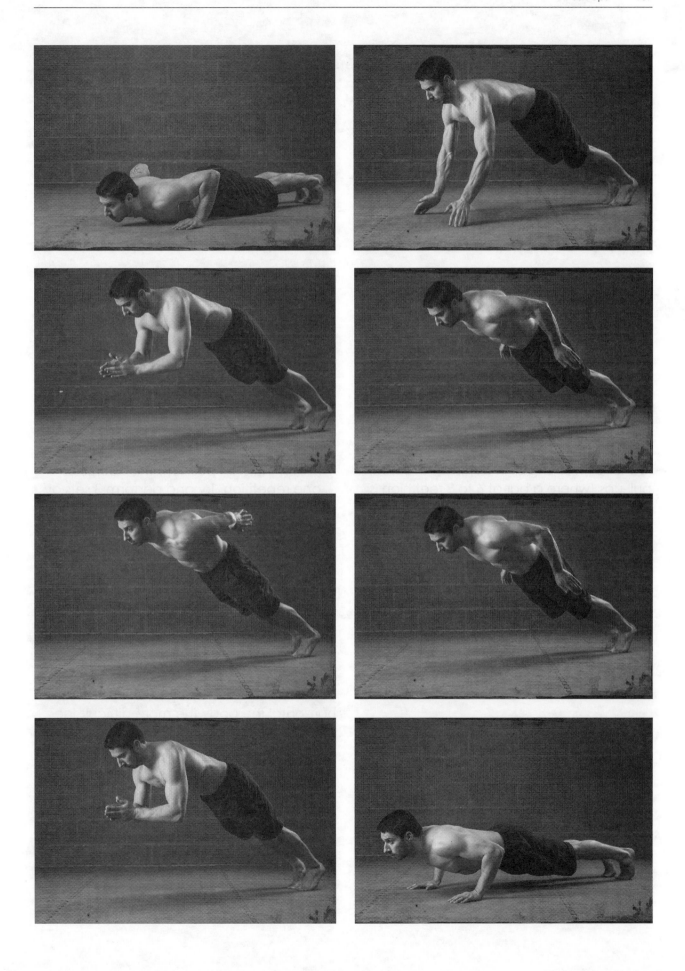

Now that we have looked at the different types of push-ups, it is time to look at the exercise that can be considered the partner to them, the pull-up. Pull-ups are, to my mind, the best upper body exercises ever. They have been used for centuries to build strong, functional physiques. They are also extremely simple in nature, can be learned relatively easily, and there are many different variations that can be used to build really extreme levels of strength. To start with we will look at building a base level, and then progress on to more and more advanced movements.

Rows

The first pulling exercise that we are going to look at is the row. Although not really a pull-up, it uses the same muscle groups as the pull-up, but it is a lot easier to perform than the proper versions. This makes it ideal for those of you who have never trained with pull-ups before, or those who have a low level of strength. In contrast to actual pull-ups (where a bar at 6 to 8 feet high is ideal), for rows you will need a bar or other object that sits around waist height. If you are a member of a gym then you can use the squat rack, smith machine, etc. If you are not a member of a gym, then you will have to use any everyday objects available to you, e.g. a table, or a bar suspended on the back of two chairs, etc. Rows can also be performed on gymnastic rings or suspension trainers with great success.

1. Grab the bar or object you are using with an overhand grip, with your hands shoulder width apart.

2. Position your body underneath the bar and place your heels on the ground.

3. Starting with your arms completely straight, pull your chest towards the bar, whilst keeping an imaginary straight line through the shoulders, hips, knees, and ankles. You should pivot around your feet or heels.

4. Once your chest reaches the bar or is level with your hands, straighten your arms and lower your body until you reach the start position. This counts as one repetition. Try and perform 3 sets of 10 repetitions to begin with, and progress from there.

Teaching Points

We can alter the difficulty of the row using the same method as that for the push-up exercises. The angle of the body in the row determines the challenge, where the more horizontal the body the more difficult the exercise, and the more vertical the body the easier the exercise. So to make the movement more or less challenging, either make your body more horizontal or more vertical. As you become stronger, simply move the body into a more horizontal position. Once you can perform rows with a completely horizontal body, then you should move onto the next exercise in this section, the chin-up.

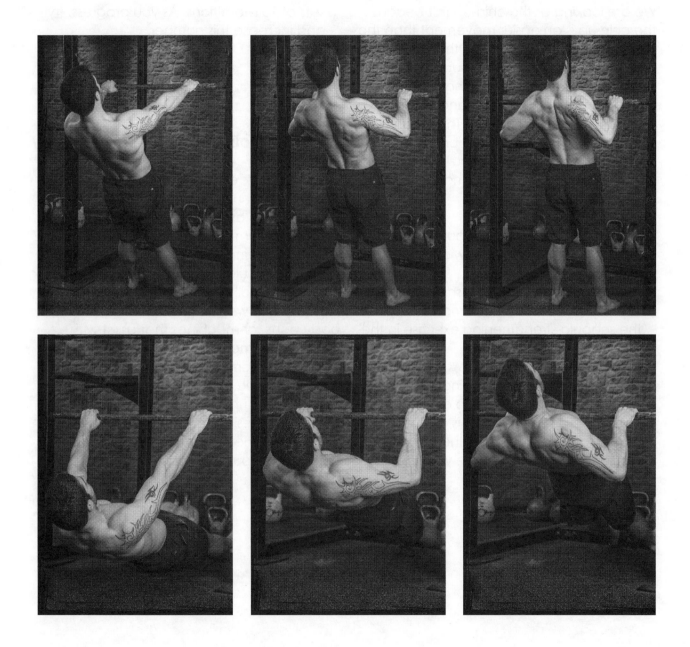

Chin-up

Once you have built up some basic strength with bodyweight rows, it is time to begin working with your entire bodyweight. We are looking at the chin-up first because the chin-up is an easier movement than the pull-up, primarily because of the way the hands grip the bar. In a chin-up the hands are in an underhand, or supinated grip, whereas in the pull-up the hands are in an overhand, or pronated grip. This means that the chin-up involves the biceps and chest much more than the pull-up, which is why the majority of people find them easier to perform than the pull-up.

1. Grasp a pull-up bar with your hands in an underhand grip, shoulder width apart.

2. Before you begin the pull, shrug your shoulders down first, as demonstrated in the scapula strengthening exercise in the mobility section.

3. Making sure you are hanging freely with your elbows locked, pull up as far as you can, ideally until your chin is above the bar or your chest touches the bar. Try not to use momentum or move your legs to help you.

4. From this top position, lower yourself down to a dead hang. This counts as one repetition. You should aim to perform 3 sets of 10 repetitions. As you progress, try and increase this number.

Teaching Points

Many people, even those who have trained for a number of years, struggle with chin-ups and pull-ups. The movement relies on a number of muscle groups being strong, including the hands and grip, forearms, shoulders, back, and core. It also requires all of these parts to work in unison. This is why machines that isolate body parts, or machines that assist with whole body movements, never help to improve performance. The chin-up is a great example of a multi-joint exercise, and simply cannot be trained for using isolation exercises or resistance machines. Next, you will see two methods you can use to help to increase your strength in the chin-up, the negative chin-up and static holds.

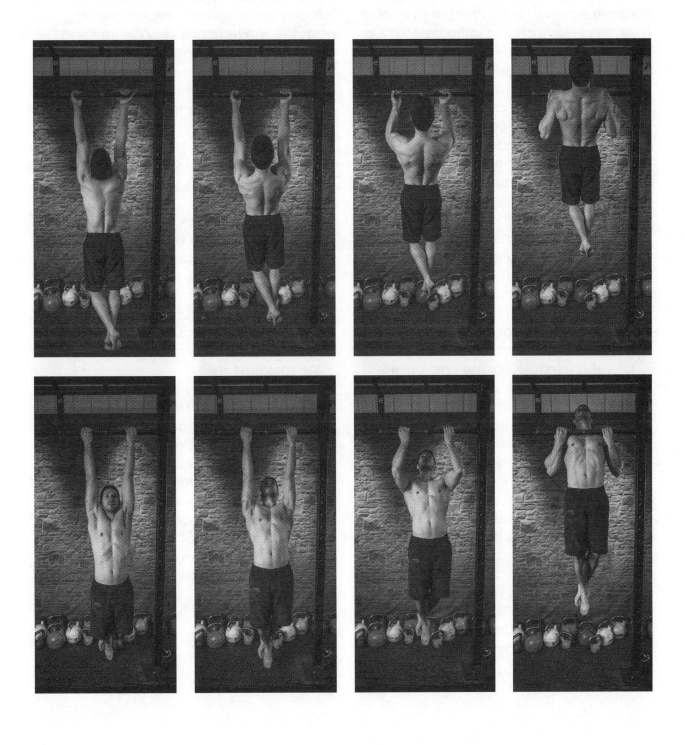

Negative Chin-up

Although many people try and perform easier exercises to build strength to enable them to perform chin-ups, the best way to progress with the chin-up is to actually do chin-ups! If your strength level is not yet high enough to pull your own weight towards the bar however, we can use a method called negative chin-ups, or **negatives**, to put the muscles under enough stress to elicit some serious strength gains. Negatives are also known as **eccentric** contractions, which simply means that the muscle being used will be contracting and getting longer (this is exactly the opposite of a **concentric**, or positive contraction, in which the muscle is contracting and getting shorter).

As the human body is strongest in the negative phase, it makes it useful for building strength when the positive phase is not yet attainable. For the chin-up, this simply means that we will not be pulling ourselves up towards the bar; instead, we will be beginning from the top of the movement, where the chin is over the bar, and lowering ourselves down to the bottom position as slowly as possible.

Negatives can be used as long as necessary or until you develop the strength to pull up towards the bar. Do not worry that you will not be practicing actually pulling up; if you stick with negatives, ultimately everything will click and you will simply be able to perform the exercise starting with straight arms.

You should not be aiming to perform lots and lots of sets and repetitions. Any negative movement is very demanding on the body, so the stresses and strains on the tendons and ligaments are very high. Four sets of 1 or 2 repetitions should be more than adequate to elicit some serious strength gains.

1. Grasp a pull-up bar with an underhand grip, with the hands shoulder width apart.

2. Now stand on a box or step below the pull-up bar you are using. Bend your legs and jump into the air, aiming to get your chin well above the bar as you do so.

3. Once you have your chin over the bar, begin to pull as hard as you can. The idea is to "catch" yourself at the top of the movement.

4. From this top position, lower yourself down as slowly as you physically can. Squeeze your muscles as hard as possible to generate maximum tension in those parts of the body being used.

5. Keep lowering yourself down until you reach the bottom of the movement, with the arms straight and elbows locked out. Now drop off the bar. This counts as one repetition.

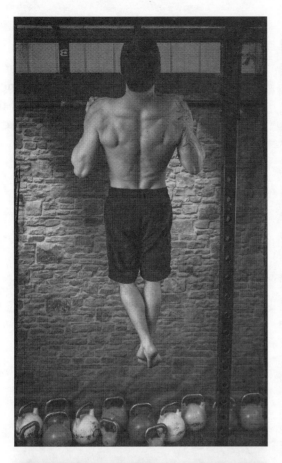

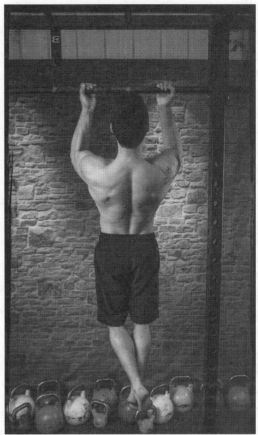

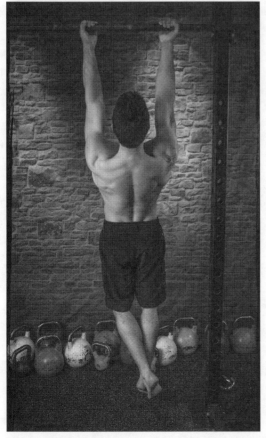

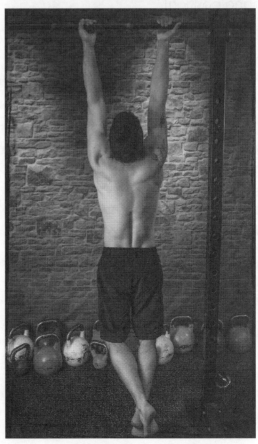

Static Holds

The second method that you can use to build strength is to work with static holds. These are where the muscles will be contracting but staying the same length. A powerlifter was quoted as once saying, "What's the heaviest weight you can lift? One that you can't lift!" What he meant by this is that any exercises where the muscles are contracting but not shortening or lengthening build huge amounts of strength.

For us, we want to look at a minimum of three elbow positions to get the greatest benefit from using static holds. These are when the elbow is as closed as possible (so when your chin is over the bar), when the elbow is at 90 degrees (so when you are halfway through the movement), and when the elbow is only slightly closed (so when you have just started to pull from the dead hang position).

1. Grab a pull-up bar with an underhand or supinated grip.

2. From here, get into the position that you wish to hold. For holding the top position with the elbows almost completely closed, you can use a box to jump into the top position. To hold the position with the elbows at 90 degrees you can also use a box, but just not jump as high. For the bottom position you can simply begin from a dead hang and then pull up slightly.

3. Once you are in the position of your choice, then simply hold it for as long as possible. As soon as the angle of the elbow starts to change and you become tired, drop off the bar and rest.

Teaching Points

In terms of the sets and repetitions for this exercise, you should try and aim to hold the position for a total time of 30 seconds, in as many sets as it takes you. For example, if you can hold the position for 10 seconds, do 3 sets of these.

Also, some angles are easier to hold than others. It goes without saying that the angles you struggle with the most are the ones that you should be training the most. As with the negative chin-ups, spend as much time with these as you need to be able to perform them properly.

Pull-up

One you have mastered the chin-up, you can move onto the pull-up. As I explained previously, the pull-up differs from the chin-up in its hand position only. For the pull-up we use an overhand or pronated grip, which has the effect of opening up the chest and lessening the ability of the biceps to help out with the pull. This means that the majority of the movement must come from the back, more specifically the latissimus dorsi, and commonly known as the lats. These are the big wing-like muscles that make up most of the upper back. Pull-ups are essential if you are aiming to have that 'V" shape back that everyone wants. They must also be mastered if you are ever to develop real pulling strength, especially if you wish to move onto the more advanced pulling exercises like the front lever and muscle-up.

The pull-up is also the second foundational exercise that we have come across, which means that this movement must be perfected before much progress can be made with the more advanced exercises in the book. See Program 1 (Fundamental Five) in Part V to see exactly what standards are required and how to train as a beginner.

1. Grasp a pull-up bar with an overhand or pronated grip. Your hands should be about shoulder width apart, or slightly wider.

2. Hang with your arms completely straight. This is also known as the dead hang position. Do not get into the habit of starting with your elbows slightly bent, as this will hinder your progress later on.

3. Before you start the pull, shrug your shoulders down first, as demonstrated in the scapula strengthening exercise in the mobility section. Then pull yourself towards the bar, keeping your legs straight. The aim is to get the chest touching the bar or the chin over the bar. Do not swing or lift your knees to make it easier.

4. From the top position lower yourself down to the start position, with completely straight arms again. This counts as one repetition. You should be aiming to perform 3 to 4 sets of 8 to 10 repetitions.

Teaching Points

Again, if you struggle to perform the movement as described, then spend some time training using negative pull-ups and static holds until your strength increases and you are able to perform the movement properly. As negative pull-ups are very taxing on the body, it is not advised to perform lots of repetitions in one go. When I work with negative pull-ups I prefer to keep the number of sets high but the number of repetitions low. For example, I often perform 5 or 6 sets of 3 repetitions, as this gives enough volume to have an effect, but not too many that my form suffers towards the end of the workout.

Shown overleaf is the overhand grip position. The top two pictures show the hand position with thumbs over the bar, which can be more comfortable for some people. The bottom two pictures show a hand position with the thumbs wrapped under the bar. Experiment to see which one you prefer.

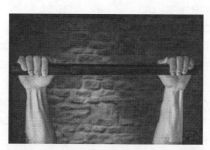

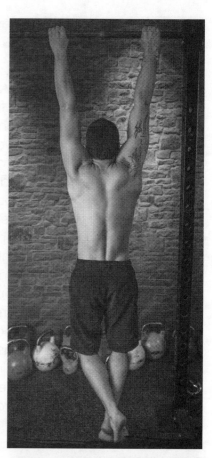

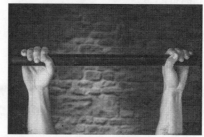

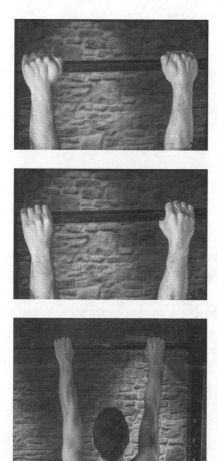

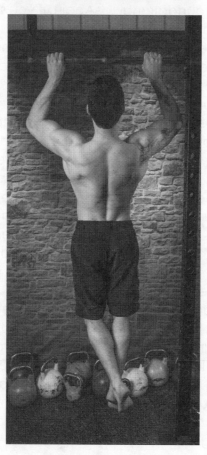

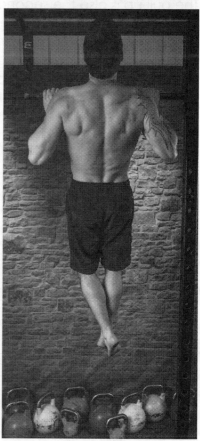

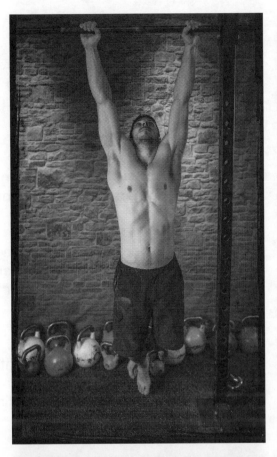
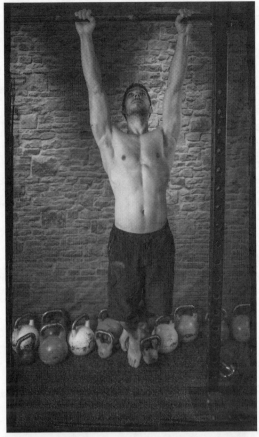
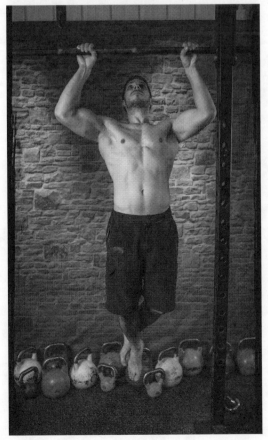
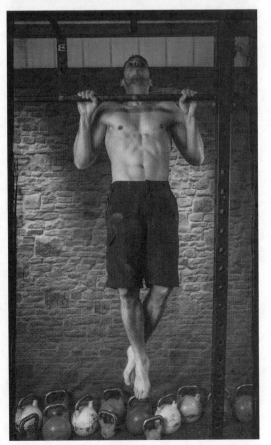

Wide Grip Pull-up

Once pull-ups become easier, we can widen the grip to make the exercise more challenging. The wide grip pull-up is excellent for targeting the latissimus dorsi muscles of the back more and, as the name suggests, this exercise uses a wider grip than the pull-up. The technique for this exercise is exactly the same as for the pull-up, except that the hands are placed on the bar as wide apart as is comfortable. The action of widening the grip means that the muscles used in pulling are stretched out even more, so that the movement is more difficult to complete, which in turn builds more strength.

1. Grasp a pull-up bar with an overhand grip. Try and position your hands as wide apart as you can.

2. Hang with your arms completely straight. Do not get into the habit of starting with your elbows slightly bent, as this will hinder your progress later on.

3. Before you start the pull, shrug your shoulders down, as demonstrated in the scapula strengthening exercise in the mobility section.

4. Pull yourself towards the bar, keeping your legs straight. Try and get your chin well above the bar. Do not swing or lift your knees to make it easier.

5. From the top position lower yourself down to the start position. This counts as one repetition. Again try and aim to perform 3 to 4 sets of 8 to 10 repetitions.

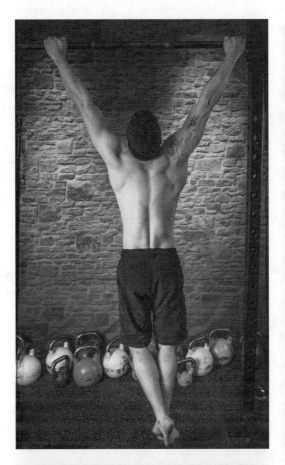

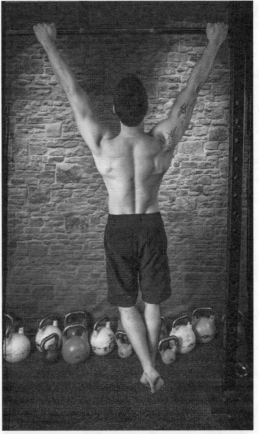

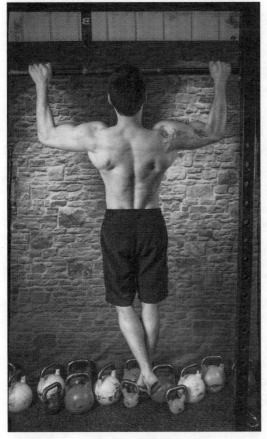

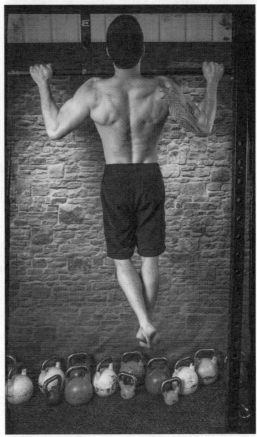

Close Grip Pull-up

Once you are familiar with the chin-up and pull-up, it is time to start incorporating other types of pull-up into your training, both to introduce variation and to hit the muscles of the body from different angles and place it under different demands. The second pull-up variation that we are going to look at is the close grip pull-up, where the hands are closer together on the bar. This really makes the biceps work more than they would in a normal pull-up, and are a fun and useful addition to your pull-up training.

1. Grasp a pull-up bar with an overhand grip. Try and position your hands as close as you can.

2. Hang with your arms completely straight. Do not get into the habit of starting with your elbows slightly bent, as this will hinder your progress later on.

3. Before you start the pull, shrug your shoulders down, as demonstrated in the scapula strengthening exercise in the mobility section.

4. Pull yourself towards the bar, keeping your legs straight. Try and get your chin well above the bar. Do not swing or lift your knees to make it easier.

5. From the top position lower yourself down to the start position. This counts as one repetition. Try and perform 3 sets of 8 to 10 repetitions.

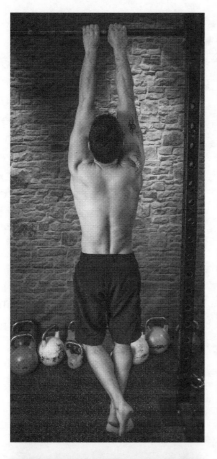
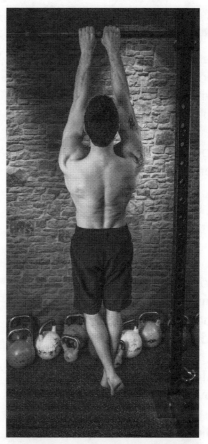
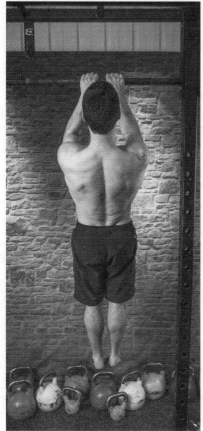
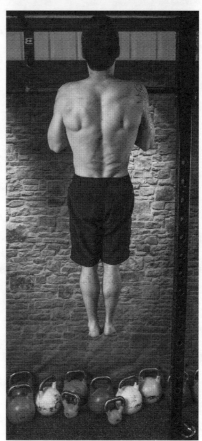

Behind the Neck Pull-up

The behind the neck pull-up is another very good variation on the pull-up, and is excellent for hitting the target muscles from a different angle. You will probably find this variation quite difficult, as the muscles used for pulling will be at a slight disadvantage due to the orientation of the body.

1. Grasp a pull-up bar with an overhand grip. Your hands should be shoulder width apart.

2. Hang with your arms completely straight. Do not get into the habit of starting with your elbows slightly bent, as this will hinder your progress later on.

3. Before you start the pull, shrug your shoulders down, as demonstrated in the scapula strengthening exercise in the mobility section.

4. Pull yourself towards the bar, keeping your legs straight. Push your head forwards and pull your shoulders blades back. You should aim to get the trapezius muscles, commonly known as the traps (the muscles on each side of the head and connected to the neck) as close to the bar as possible. You can see the back of my neck touching the bar in the pictures. Do not swing or lift your knees to make it easier.

5. From the top position lower yourself down to the start position. This counts as one repetition. Try and perform 3 sets of 8 to 10 repetitions.

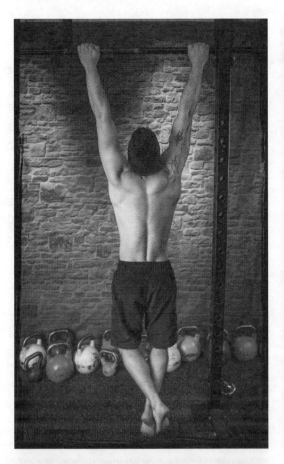

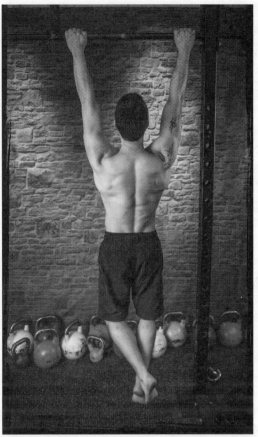

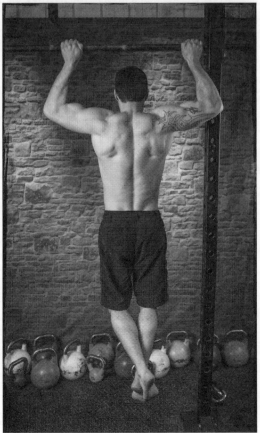

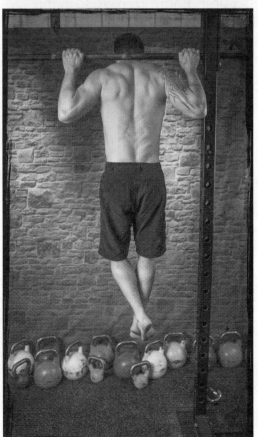

Inline Pull-up

The inline pull-up is a variation that I first came across whilst in military training. Our training team made us perform these to help with rope climbing, and I found them so effective that I carried on performing them once I had left the military. They are a kind of mixture between a pull-up and a row that we looked at earlier, and have some good carryover strength to the more difficult movements like the front lever.

1. Stand underneath a pull-up bar and grab it with the palms facing in towards each other, and make sure that they are close enough on the bar to be touching.

2. Hang with straight arms and have your head leaning back.

3. Before you begin the pull, shrug your shoulders down, as demonstrated in the scapula strengthening exercise in the mobility section.

4. From here, pull as hard as you can and attempt to get your chest touching the bar. You will have to lean back a lot to get this to happen, so it pays to relax the lower body so that it does not drift out in front of you too much.

5. Once you have pulled as high as you are able to, extend your arms again until you reach the start position. This counts as one repetition.

Teaching Points

The picture opposite shows the hand position for the inline pull-up. Ensure that your hands are as close together as possible.

In terms of sets and repetitions, try and perform 3 sets of 8 to 10 repetitions.

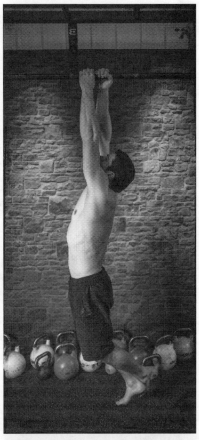

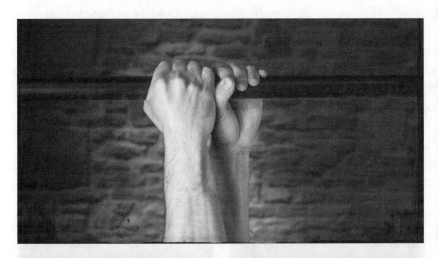

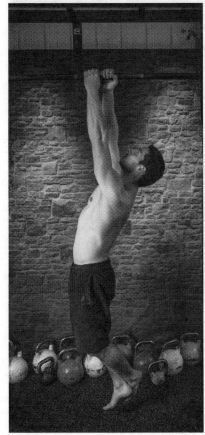

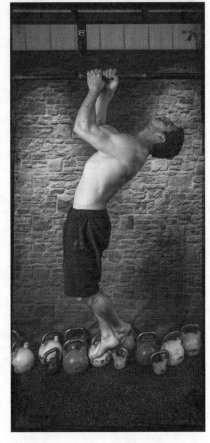

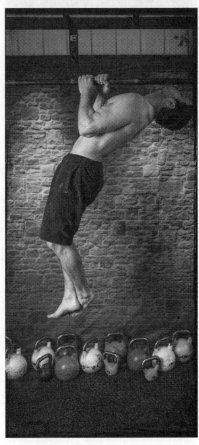

Rock Climber Pull-up

Once you have mastered the wide grip pull-up, you can start to work with the rock climber. This exercise probably did originate with actual rock climbers, as they need to be able to traverse left and right as well as straight up. The rock climber involves pulling more with one arm than the other, and will give you a small taste of what it is like to work with one-arm pull-ups, which are featured later on.

1. Grab a pull-up bar with an overhand grip, with your hands as wide apart as they are in a wide grip pull-up.

2. Before you start the pull, shrug your shoulders down, as demonstrated in the scapula strengthening exercise in the mobility section.

3. From here, pull yourself strongly to one side, so that your whole body moves towards one hand. At this point one arm will be more bent than the other and the other will be nearly straight.

4. Now lower yourself back down to the start position, and then pull yourself up towards the opposite hand. Each pull counts as one repetition. You should aim to perform 3 sets of 8 repetitions, with 4 repetitions on each side.

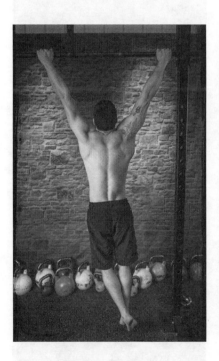
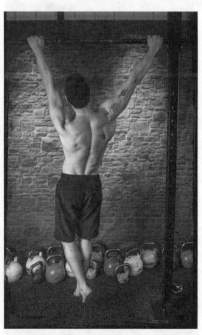
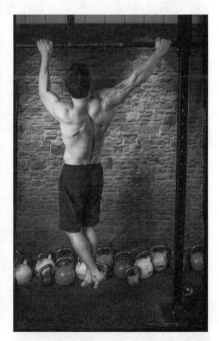

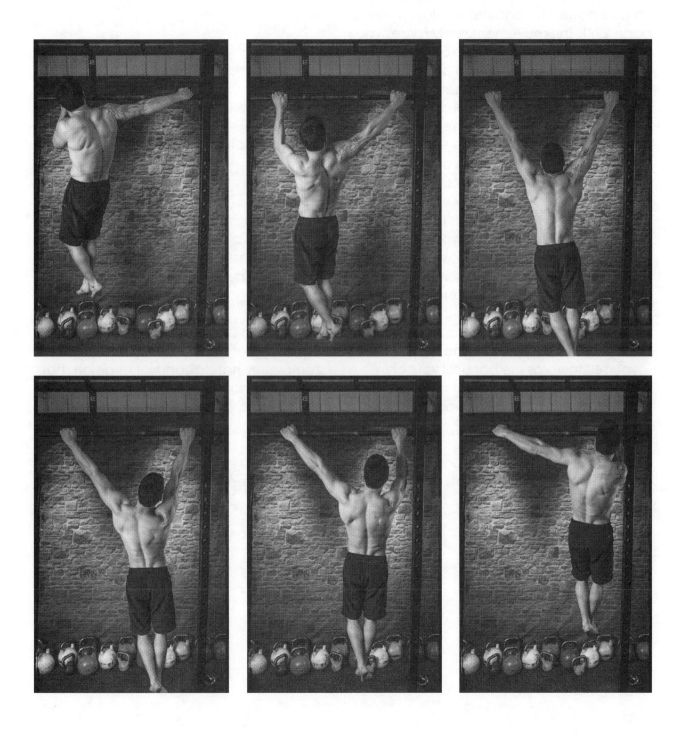

L Pull-up

The L pull-up has features of both the pull-up (see page 117) and the half lever (see page 227). This movement really forces you to use the back to pull with properly, and as the legs and core have to be held in a static position as well, it means that it is almost impossible to cheat on this exercise, as long as it is performed correctly.

1. Grab a pull-up bar with an overhand grip and hang with straight arms.

2. From here, raise up the legs until they are horizontal. Make sure that you keep the knee joints locked out. You will notice at this point that the body resembles an "L" shape, which is why the exercise has the name it does.

3. Holding this position with the legs, pull yourself towards the bar until your chin reaches over it. Notice that my legs stay as horizontal as possible throughout the whole movement.

4. Then lower yourself down until you reach the start position. This counts as one repetition.

Teaching Points

If you cannot either perform the leg raise or hold the legs in an "L" position, spend time with the leg raise and the half lever to build up strength. You can also work with the legs at an angle instead of horizontal, and then as you become stronger simply move them up.

Many people struggle to perform both the pull and the leg raise at the same time. This is completely natural, and is just a sign that your body is not strong enough to do both simultaneously. Spend more time with each separate movement and then progress when you are ready.

For sets and repetitions, you should aim to perform 3 to 4 sets of 5 to 8 repetitions.

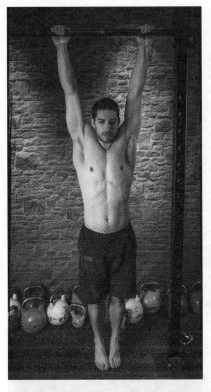
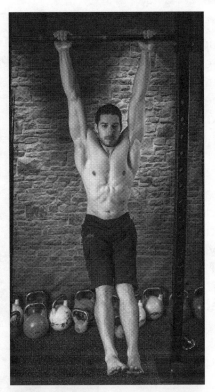
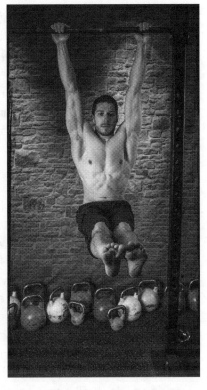

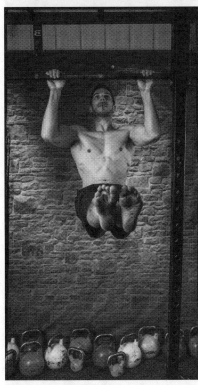
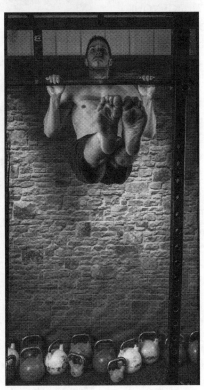

Horizontal Pull-up

Continuing with our look at different types of pull-up, the horizontal pull-up is a unique exercise that has elements of a pull-up, an inline pull-up, and a front lever. It uniquely stresses the core and has some elements of muscular control within it, which makes it a challenge to those looking for more difficult pulling exercises.

1. Grab a pull-up bar in an overhand grip, with the hands about shoulder width apart. This exercise is also particularly suited to monkey bars, or two bars that are parallel to each other. If you use this method then your hands will be gripping the bars facing in towards each other.

2. From here, pull up and back at the same time, aiming to end with your eyes facing the ceiling and your body in a horizontal position. You will need to contract your lower back, glutes, and other lower body muscles hard to make sure that your body remains horizontal.

3. Keep pulling as your body becomes horizontal, as the aim of this exercise is to get the body as close to the bar as possible.

4. Hold the horizontal position for a split second, and then lower yourself back down to the start position under control. This counts as one repetition.

Teaching Points

As the horizontal pull-up puts so much of a demand on the upper body and the core muscles, you should aim to perform 3 to 4 sets of 5 repetitions.

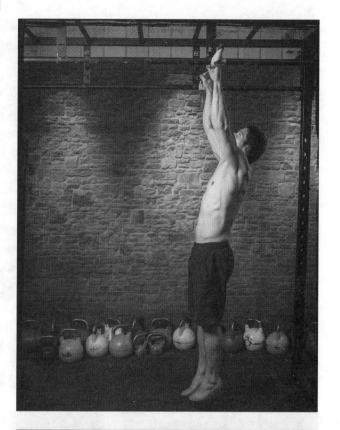

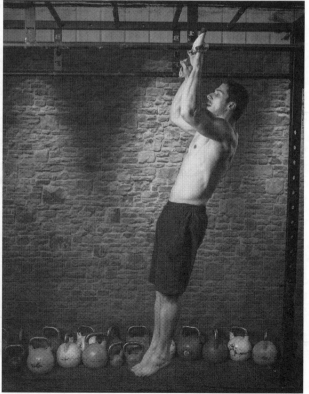

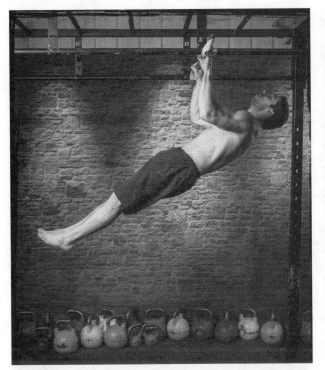

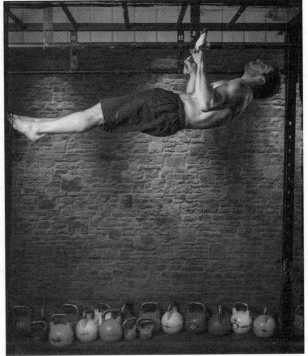

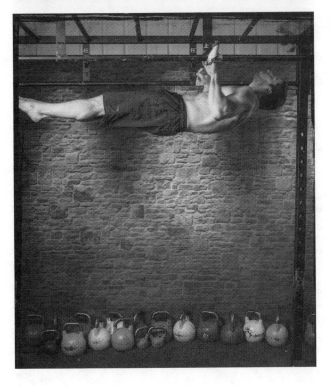

Finger Pull-up

Finger pull-ups are another exercise, like fingertip push-ups, that can help to build real hand and grip strength. As you progress with finger pull-ups you can simply reduce the number of fingers you use to make the exercise more challenging. Using chalk for this exercise is recommended.

1. Grip the bar with an underhand or overhand grip using only the fingers on each hand. As said before, you can reduce the number of fingers you use as you become stronger.

2. From a dead hang, pull up strongly until your chin reaches over the bar.

3. Lower yourself down until you reach the start position. This counts as one repetition. Try and perform 3 sets of 3 to 5 repetitions to begin with, and then increase this number as your strength increases.

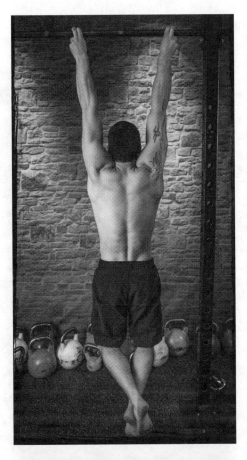
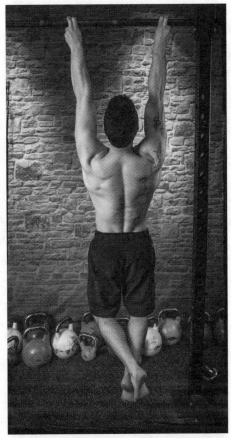
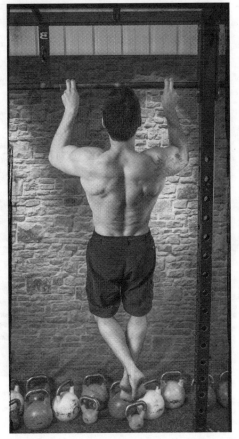
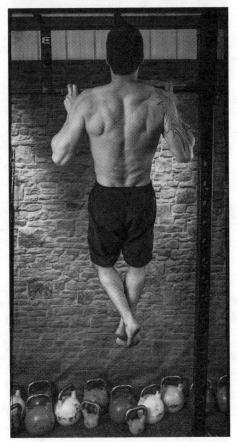

Rope/Towel Pull-up

We will look at using a rope or towel to help assist with the one-arm pull-up later on in this chapter, but we can also use the rope or towel as an actual pulling object. The rope or towel pull-up is an amazing grip strength builder, and is quite different from the other movements we have looked at so far, in that the object you are pulling on, either a rope or towel or other fabric-like object, is free to move around and is not fixed.

If you have access to a rope then this is the best tool to use, as they are normally very good to grip. Most gyms do not have ropes however, and they are not that cheap to buy. In this case it is best to use a towel or other similar piece of fabric or cloth. Simply drape the towel or cloth over the pull-up bar until both ends meet. Then you can grab this quite comfortably with both hands.

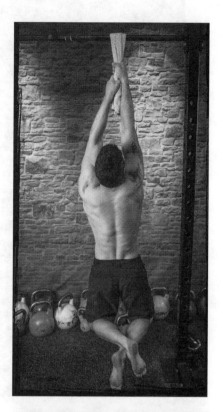

1. Grab the rope or towel with one hand on top of the other, or you can use a towel in each hand.

2. From a dead hang, pull up as far as you can. The aim is to get the hands level with the sternum (the bony plate in the middle of your chest).

3. From here, lower yourself back down to the start position. This counts as one repetition.

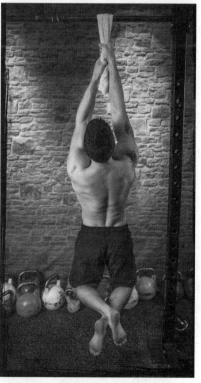

Teaching Points

Your grip strength will determine how many repetitions you can perform, so start with 3 sets of 5 repetitions and then build up from there.

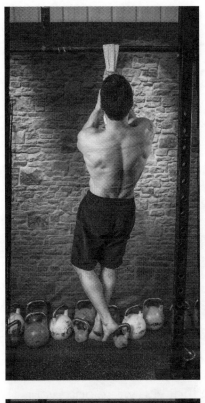
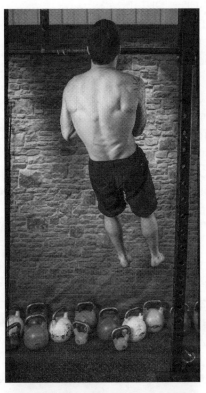
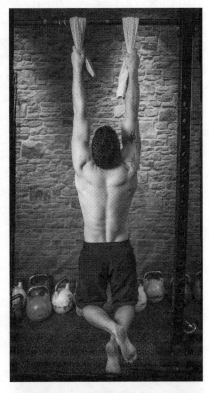
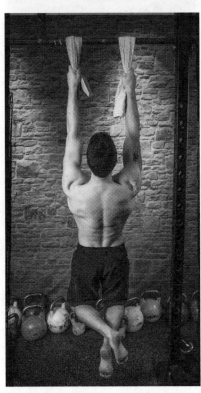
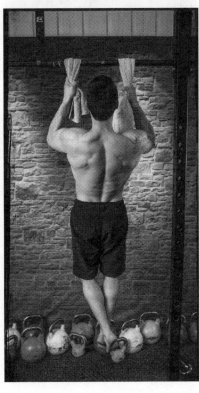
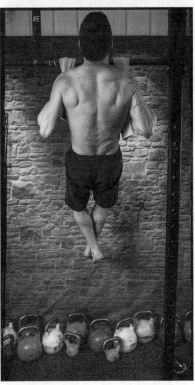

Clap Pull-up

The clap pull-up is a flashy exercise, but it is not just for show. The power needed to do this is extreme, and the exercise also builds a large amount of confidence and coordination. It goes without saying that you will need access to a pull-up bar that can take the strain of your own weight and the force that will be applied to it when you catch it. I would also recommend clearing the area behind the bar, because if you do miss the bar when you attempt to catch it, at least you will not fall onto anything.

A downside to the clap pull-up is that there is not really any way to regress the exercise, or make it easier. When you start to work with it you will just have to give it a go and see what happens.

1. Grasp a pull-up bar with an overhand grip and hang with straight arms.

2. From here, pull up as hard and as powerfully as possible, aiming to pull far past the bar.

3. As your chin becomes level with the bar, take your hands off and clap once in front of your chest. Keep your eyes on the bar at all times.

4. As soon as you have clapped, bring your hands back to the bar and catch it strongly, then lower yourself down to the start position. This counts as one repetition.

Teaching Points

Performing the clap pull-up is a great challenge, and not just because it requires a great deal of strength. The main issue you will come up against is that it requires a lot of confidence to take the hands away from the bar in the first place. To remedy this, you can perform a pull-up, but when your chin gets level with the bar, simply make your hands go light. This does not mean that you will release your grip; it simply means that you will lessen the grip for a split second. As you gain more confidence, you can start to lessen the amount that you are holding onto the bar until your hands actually come away from it. Then you can begin to gradually progress onto bringing the hands together and clapping. As with any difficult exercise, start small and progress gradually and you will always be successful.

As it is such a powerful movement, try to do 3 or 4 sets of 1 or 2 repetitions initially and then increase the number as you gain strength.

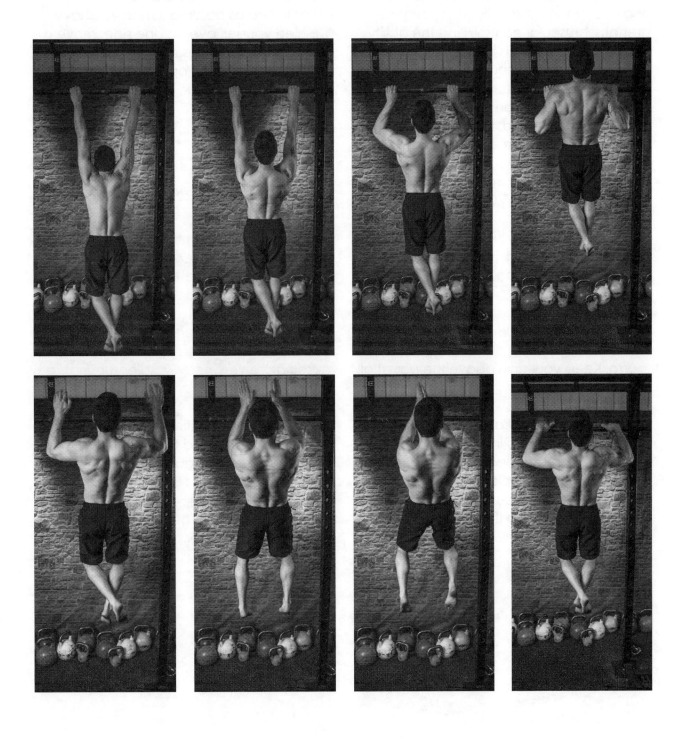

Typewriter Pull-up

The next exercise in this pull-up chapter is also one of the most difficult. It combines strength, muscular control, and the ability to generate tension in the entire upper body. The typewriter pull-up has elements of the wide grip pull-up, the rock climber, and the muscle-up, and will test your shoulder strength and, more importantly your scapula strength, to the limit.

1. Grab a pull-up bar in an overhand grip with your hands as wide apart as you can.

2. From a dead hang, pull up until your chin is above the bar and then hold the position.

3. From here, pull yourself over to one arm whilst straightening out the opposite arm. Keep your chin above the bar at all times.

4. As you move towards your pulling arm you will need to go into a half false grip with the arm that becomes straight. You can see this in the pictures opposite. This is so that you can push down hard with the straight arm, so that your chin stays above the bar.

5. The movement should be as slow and controlled as possible. Once you have pulled yourself over to one side, move yourself back to the middle of the bar and repeat on the opposite side.

Teaching Points

When first attempting this movement you will no doubt find it very difficult. I have found that getting better at the muscle-up can help with the typewriter, and improving your false grip as well. It is common to find that this movement also stresses the insides of the shoulders, or the rotator cuff musculature very heavily, so ensure not to overdo it.

The number of repetitions you can perform will be directly related to your ability to keep your shoulders above the pull-up bar. To begin with try to do 3 sets of 4 repetitions, alternating to the left and right side each time. Increase this number as you become stronger.

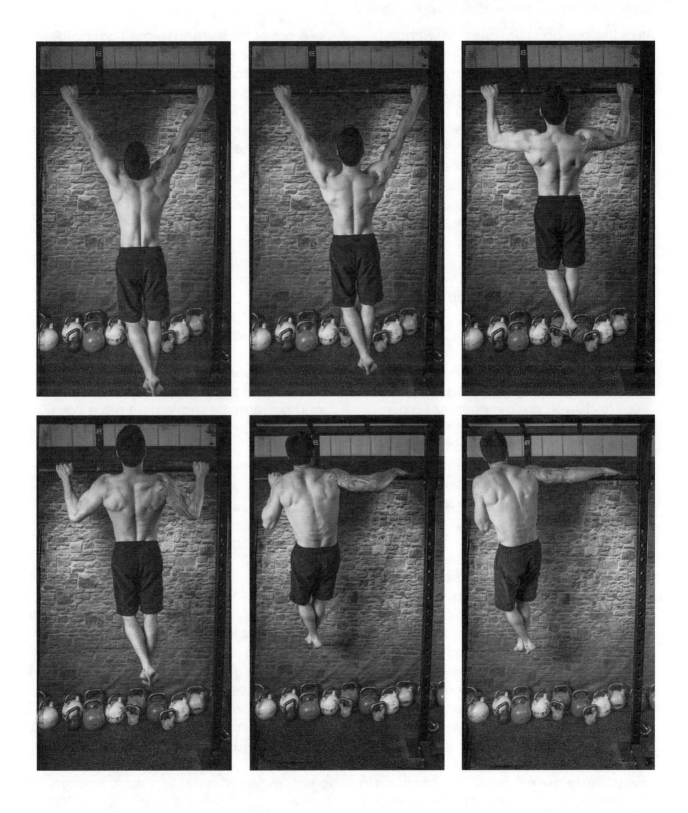

Weighted Pull-up

All of the pull-up variations that we have looked at so far have been unweighted, that is, they only use your bodyweight as the resistance. After all, this book is all about using your own bodyweight to become much stronger! However, after a time, you will have enough strength to start working with weighted versions of the pull-ups that are in this chapter. These are very useful, as the movement stays essentially the same; it is just the resistance that increases.

There are a few ways to add weight to the body and we will look at three of them here:

• The first method is to use a dumbbell or kettlebell held between the feet. This has the advantage of being easy to set up, and if you are a member of a gym, there should be plenty of dumbbells and kettlebells of varying sizes and weights available. To hold the weight, simply grab it between your feet as shown opposite, and perform the pull-up exercise of your choice.

• The second method is to use a dip belt. Again, these can be found in most gyms, and usually take the form of a neoprene or leather belt with a chain attached. You can thread the chain through the centre of weight plates, and then allow the weight to dangle between your legs where it will stay out of the way. Again perform the pull-up variation of your choice.

• The third method is to use a weighted vest. These are not really that common in commercial gyms, and the chances of your local gym having one are slim. They can be bought in certain shops or online, but unless you think you will get a lot of

use out of them, then I would not bother to purchase one. Weighted vests come in a variety of different types, but most of them use the same formula, which is a vest or jacket that fits over the upper body, with pouches of sand, water, gel, or actual metal weights used to increase or decrease the resistance. To use these, you simply put the vest on and perform the pull-up variation of your choice.

1. Choose one of the methods of adding weight as outlined previously, and hang from the bar with straight arms.

2. Now simply perform the pull-up variation of your choice.

3. As you become stronger, try to increase the amount of weight that you use, or try and perform the movement more slowly.

Teaching Points

There are a number of methods we can use in terms of the sets and repetitions that you should perform. If you are using a light weight, such as 10 kg or 20 lbs, then aim for 3 sets of 8 to 10 repetitions. If you are using a really heavy weight then it is totally fine to do only a couple repetitions for a few sets. For example, I often use 50 to 60kg, or 100 to 120lbs, and then try and do only 1 or 2 repetitions to increase my strength as much as possible.

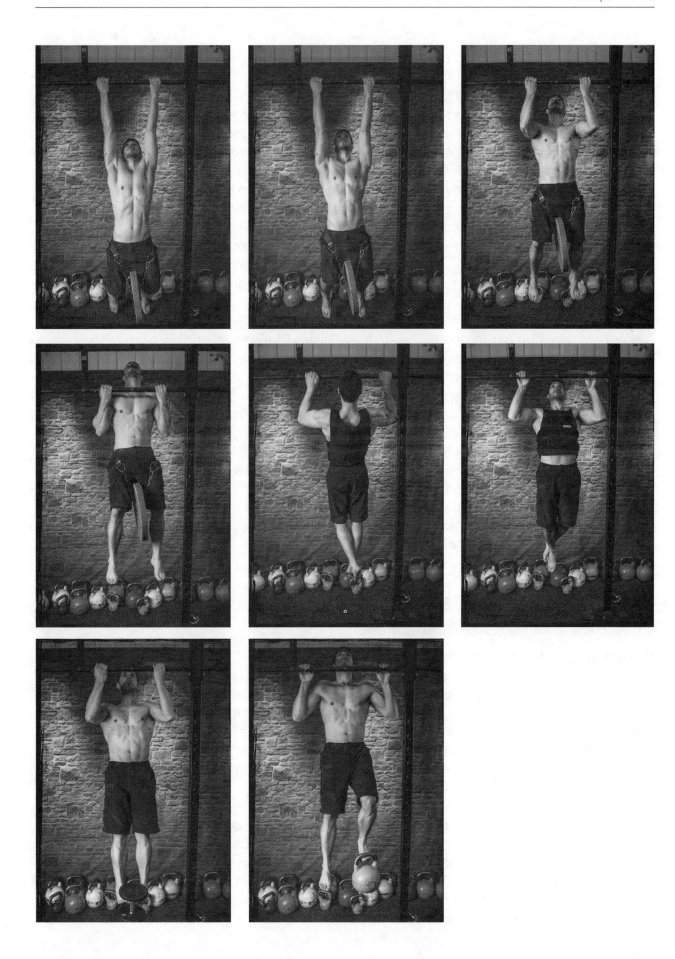

One-Arm Pull-up

The one-arm pull-up is perhaps the Holy Grail for most people that start calisthenic training. Performing a strict one-arm pull-up can take years of dedicated effort, which is shown by the very few people who can actually perform one. This movement will place an extreme demand on your entire upper body and core. Take your time progressing with this exercise. Even if you are at an advanced level, it will take you anywhere in the region of six months to two years to accomplish.

The one-arm pull-up is also one of the few unilateral exercises that are available to us, the others being the one-arm push-up and the single-leg squat. These unilateral exercises are particularly challenging, but the reward in terms of strength and athletic ability are well worth the investment.

Some prefer to perform the one-arm pull-up with an underhand or supinated grip, and there are others who prefer to use an overhand or pronated grip. My personal preference is to use an underhand or supinated grip, but that is simply my personal preference, and is not necessarily the best way for you to do them. The best idea is to experiment with hand positions and see which you prefer, or alternatively, try and train to be able to do them with both hand positions.

As the one-arm pull-up is such a demanding exercise, it is not possible for the vast majority of people to simply jump straight in and start training it. Therefore, I have broken the movement down into five stages that should enable most people to achieve a one-arm pull-up.

1. Finger assisted one-arm pull-up
2. Towel/rope assisted one-arm pull-up
3. Negative one-arm pull-up
4. Static holds
5. One-arm pull-up

Finger Assisted One-Arm Pull-up

The first stage in learning the one-armed pull-up is to use the other arm for assistance. This acts to place less of a demand on the pulling arm so that you can gradually increase your strength. To train for the one-armed pull-up using your other arm for assistance, we can simply grab the bar using fewer fingers on the assisting hand. The fewer fingers you use, the harder the movement will become resulting in a stronger pulling arm. Start out using four fingers and no thumb, and then progress to using three fingers, two fingers, and so on. Practice with both hands equally to ensure strength imbalances do not occur.

1. Grab the bar using an underhand grip with the pulling arm and using only four fingers with the assisting arm. The assisting arm can be in either an overhand or underhand grip, depending on your personal preference.

2. Making sure you are hanging freely pull your scapula down as described in the mobility section. Pull hard with the main arm until your chin reaches over the bar.

3. As you pull yourself up, only use the assisting arm as much as you need to. Obviously, the less you use it the more challenging the movement will be to perform.

4. From here, lower yourself down until you reach the start position. This counts as one repetition.

Teaching Points

As you become stronger with this movement, you can reduce the number of fingers that grip the bar with the assisting arm. Obviously, the fewer fingers you use will reduce the amount of assistance your arm can give. Keep progressing like this until you are only using one finger on the assisting arm.

As for sets and repetitions, the purpose of this exercise is to build as much strength as possible. This means that you should only be doing 3 or 4 sets of 3 to 5 repetitions. Any more than this and the exercise will not be building enough strength.

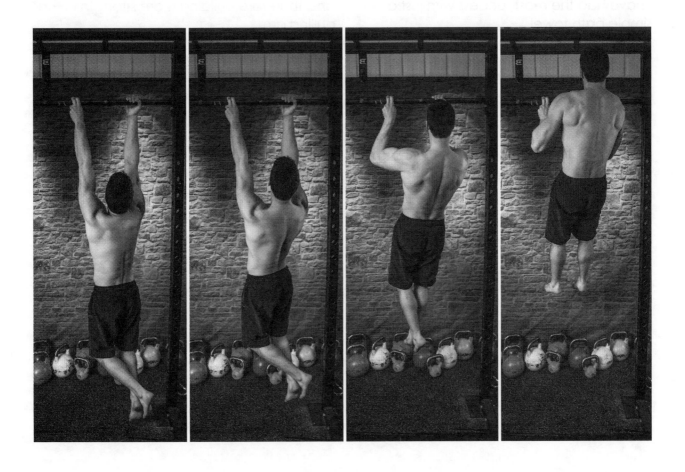

Rope/Towel Assisted One-Arm Pull-up

The next stage in learning the one-arm pull-up is the towel or rope assisted method. The idea is to grab the towel or rope with the assisting hand and use that to help with the movement. To begin with you should grab the towel or rope high up, as close to the bar as possible. As you become stronger simply grab the towel or rope lower down. This will lessen the amount of assistance that you can give yourself and make the exercise more challenging. Keep progressing like this until you are ready for the next stage.

You will obviously need a rope or a towel for this movement (or some other object that you can hang over the bar and use to hold onto). Some gyms have ropes, but I have had the most success with just a simple bath towel.

1. Grasp the pull-up bar with one hand in an underhand grip. Position the towel/rope over the pull-up bar, about shoulder width away from the pulling hand.

2. Grab the rope/towel with the assisting hand as high up as you can manage.

3. Make sure that you are hanging freely, and then start to pull hard with the pulling arm. Only give as much assistance from the assisting arm as is needed. Keep pulling until your chin reaches over the pull-up bar.

4. From this top position lower yourself back down to the start position. This counts as one repetition.

Teaching Points

As you become stronger with this variation, you can simply grab the rope or towel further down. This will make it more difficult for that arm to assist with the movement, and therefore building more strength in the pulling arm.

As for sets and repetitions, again, the purpose of this exercise is to build as much strength as possible. This means that you should only be doing 3 or 4 sets of 3 to 5 repetitions. Any more than this and the exercise will not be building enough strength.

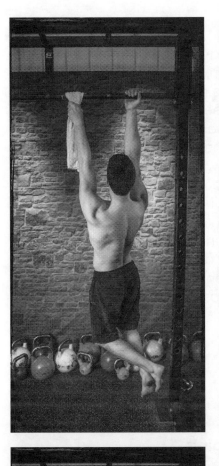
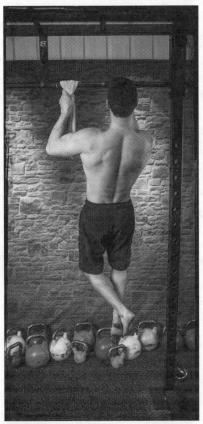
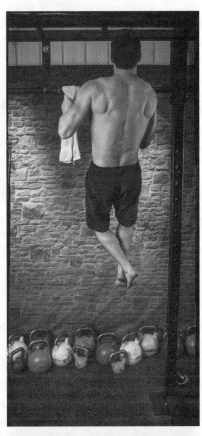

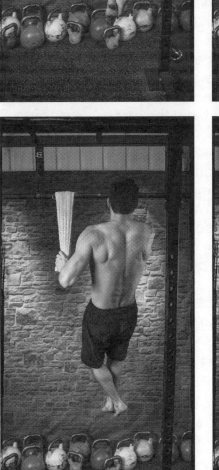
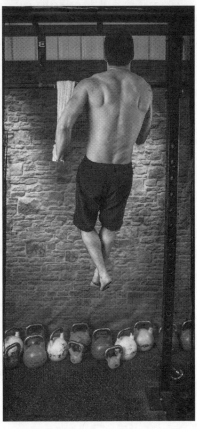

Negative One-Arm Pull-up

Once you have practiced these first two methods, it is time to move onto perhaps the best method at building strength for the one-arm pull-up, which is the negative one-arm pull-up. As the name suggests, this method uses the negative phase of the movement to build strength in the target muscles. This method is the same as the negative chin-up on page 114, in that you will start at the top of the movement, then lower yourself down as slowly as possible, trying to generate as much tension in the muscles as you are able to. This, as you might imagine, is extremely taxing on the body, so a low number of sets and repetitions should be performed at first, just until you are able to deal with the volume.

1. Grasp the bar with the target arm in an underhand grip and the assisting arm in an overhand grip. Your hands should be about shoulder width apart, but this point is not too important.

2. From here, use a box or platform to standing on and help to jump above the bar, or pull yourself over it. Whichever method you use, all that you need to do at this stage is get your chin over the bar into the top position of the pull-up.

3. From this top position, release the bar with the assisting arm. Make sure that you generate as much tension in the body as you can at this point. This is so that your pull will be stronger.

4. After you have released the bar with the assisting arm, slowly start to lower yourself down to the ground. Again, making a fist with your free hand can help to generate the much-needed tension in the body to assist with the pull. You can see me doing this to help with the movement. Also, you can raise your legs into an "L" position to help make the exercise easier.

5. Keep lowering yourself down until your pulling arm becomes completely straight. Then you can drop off the bar. This counts as one repetition.

Teaching Points

Because of the high intensity of this exercise, I would recommend performing 3 to 5 sets of 1 repetition on each arm. The demand placed on your tendons and other connective tissues is extreme, and your body will need time to gain strength. If you feel any pain in the elbows, then take plenty of rest and decrease the intensity and frequency of your one-arm pull-up training. It is highly likely that you will get some form of tendonitis in the elbows when training for the one-arm pull-up, so take a rest and allow them to recover.

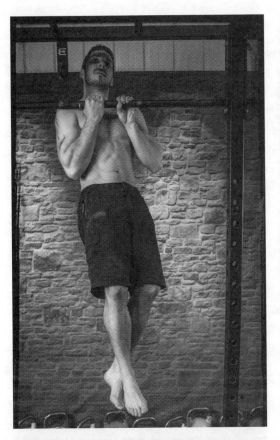

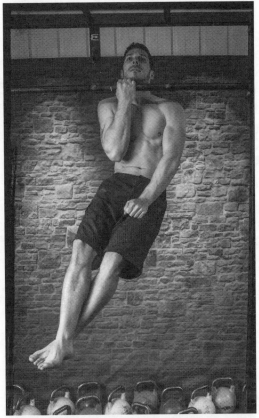

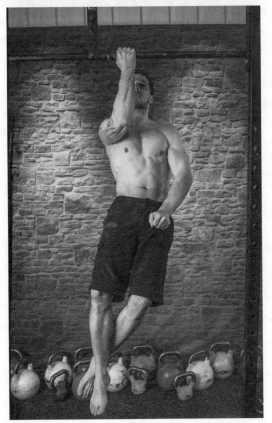

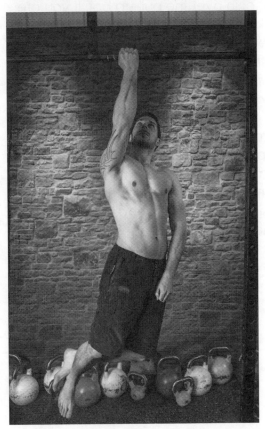

Static Holds

Before attempting the full one-arm pull up, we use static holds to build strength in the various angles of the arm. There are of course many different angles that occur in the elbow when moving through a pull-up, but we can narrow it down to three; a very closed angle at the top of the movement (where the chin is over the bar), a 90-degree angle in the elbow, and a position where the elbow is nearly straight. Working with all three of these angles will help to build huge strength throughout the whole movement.

1. Grab the pull-up bar with an underhand grip with one hand and an overhand grip with the other.

2. From here, pull yourself into the position that you want to work on. If this is the top position with a closed elbow, then pull your chin over the pull-up bar. If you are working with a 90-degree bend in the elbow, then pull yourself to this position. If it is the bottom position with only a slightly bent elbow, then pull yourself up only very slightly.

3. From these positions, let go with the supporting arm and try to hold yourself for as long as possible without bending your arm. To generate as much muscular tension as possible, clench your free hand into a fist and squeeze all of your muscle groups as tightly as possible.

4. Hold this position for as long as you can, and then when your elbow starts to bend, simply drop off, change arms, and repeat the process.

Teaching Points

With the static holds, you will want to work with all three degrees of bend in the elbow to ensure that you develop strength in all of the right places. If you find that you are weak in one particular angle, then it is perfectly fine to spend longer with that hold than others. Ultimately, static holds are simply another way to increase your strength in the run up to performing a proper one-arm chin-up. As before, with static holds you will want to try and build up to a total hold time of around 30 seconds for each position. For example, if you can only hold the movement for 5 seconds, then you would need to complete 6 sets to equal the 30-second total.

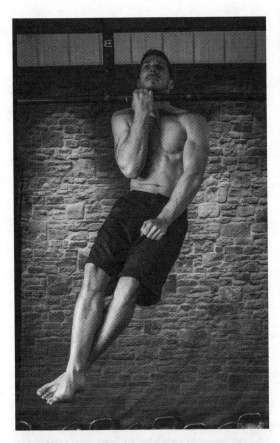

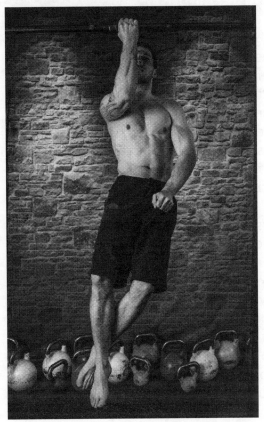

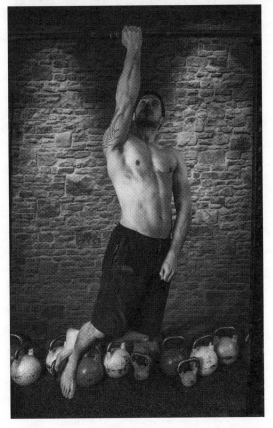

One-Arm Pull-up

Once you have trained with the assisted and negative variations long enough, you can attempt the unassisted version. There should come a time when your negative one-arm pull-ups become very, very slow, and your static holds become easier, which means that you will not be far away from performing a proper one-arm pull-up, with no assistance.

1. Grasp a pull-up bar with one hand in an under- or overhand grip.

2. Making sure you are hanging freely pull down with your scapula as described in the mobility section. This is the action that initiates the pull. If you struggle to stop yourself swinging and rotating, then simply spend time trying to control your shoulder stability in the bottom position.

3. From here, start to pull as hard as you can. Try clenching the fist of the free hand and raising the legs into an "L" position. This will help to generate muscular tension, which is vital for success in performing these higher-level exercises. Keep pulling until your chin goes over the bar, or your shoulder touches the bar.

4. Then lower yourself down until you reach the start position and your arm is locked out. This counts as one repetition.

Teaching Points

In terms of repetitions, simply perform as many as you can. This is likely to be a very low number, such as 3 sets of 1 repetition on each arm initially.

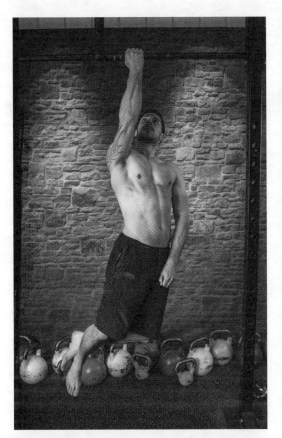

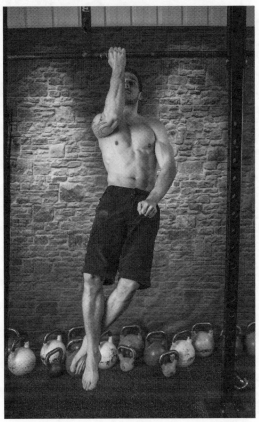

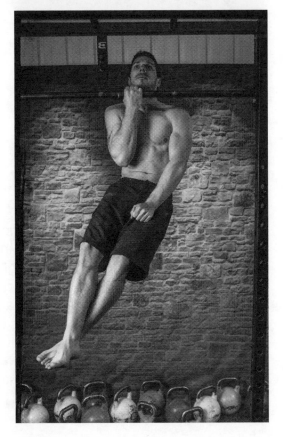

Dips are the second group of pushing and pressing exercises that we are going to look at, and are a good movement for targeting the triceps, or the back of the upper arm. All pushing and pressing movements involve the triceps heavily, and if you want big arms then these are the muscles to train. There are not as many dip variations as we have looked at for the push-up exercises, but they are a very valuable part of calisthenic training. I once heard someone refer to dips as the upper body equivalent of the squat, and I think that they were right. The dips will help to develop not just the triceps, but also the shoulders and the chest, and can be made much more difficult by simply adding weight to them.

The equipment required for the exercises in this chapter are a box or other suitable platform, access to dip bars, and once you progress onto weighted dips, a dip belt or some form of additional weight.

Box Dip

The box dip is the starting point for the dip exercises, and should be achievable even for those who have not trained before or who have a low level of strength. You will need some sort of platform or box on which to place your hands, such as an aerobic step, a chair, the end of your bed, or even a set of stairs—just ensure that the platform is sturdy and will support your weight.

1. Place your hands on the platform with your fingers facing forwards.

2. Position your legs out in front of you, balance on your heels and keep your knees locked.

3. From here, bend your elbows and allow your butt to move towards the ground. Keep your back close to the box to enable a greater range of motion. Keep bending the elbows until you reach the ground, or as far as your flexibility allows. Note that my back stays close to the box at all times, and does not drift too far away from it.

4. From the bottom position, push up hard until your elbows become straight again. This counts as one repetition.

Teaching Points

If you find the above method too difficult, then simply bend the knees to make the movement easier. This puts more weight onto the lower body and allows strength to be built in a progressive manner. As your strength increases, straighten the legs until you can perform the exercise properly.

You should be aiming to do 3 to 4 sets of 8 to 12 repetitions.

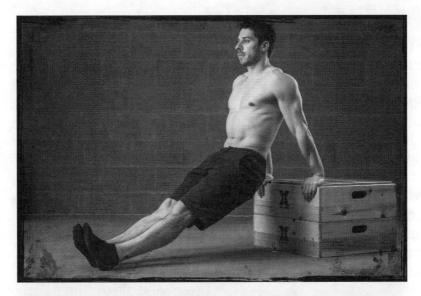

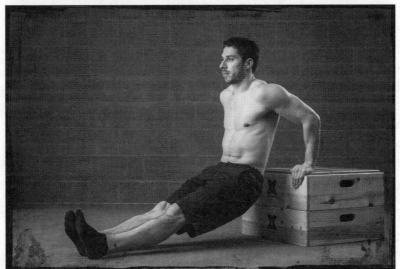

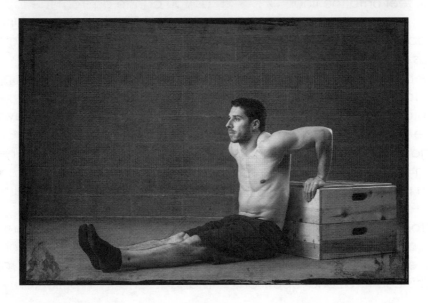

Triceps Dip

Once you have spent some time with the box dip you should be ready to move onto the proper movement; the triceps dip. This is much more difficult than the box dip, so take your time and only push your body as far as it can go. This movement is also one of the foundational exercises discussed at the beginning of this part of the book. This means that it is vital that you perfect this movement before moving on to the more advanced exercises, as dips will give you a very good grounding and solid base of strength on which you can build.

To perform the triceps dip you will need to use a set of dip bars. You can find them in any gym, or you can find versions built for home use. You can also use the backs of two chairs facing each other, but this is obviously less safe than using proper equipment built for the purpose. Whatever you use, just make sure that it is sturdy and can take your weight.

1. Grasp the bars with your palms facing inwards. Straighten your arms and get into a comfortable position: if necessary, cross your ankles behind you to avoid dropping your feet onto the floor.

2. Bend your elbows and lower yourself down as far as you can, pausing at the bottom of the movement. You may find that you start to lean forwards slightly, but this is fine. You can see that my range of motion is quite large, but do not worry if you cannot go this low initially. Just go as far as you can and increase the range of motion as you progress.

3. From this bottom position push yourself up until you reach the start position. Lock out your elbows at the top of the movement. This counts as one repetition.

Teaching Points

Many people have trouble with the triceps dip, simply because you are effectively carrying your entire body weight on your upper body. Also, the learning curve from the box dip to the triceps dip is quite significant.

To remedy this and make the exercise easier, we can use a technique that has been mentioned previously, which is the use of negatives. The negative phase of the movement occurs when you are moving with gravity. For the triceps dip, this means the movement when we are lowering ourselves down towards the ground. Conversely, when we push against gravity we are performing the positive phase of the movement.

To do this, get into the first position of the triceps dip, which has you supporting your own bodyweight with straight arms. From here, bend your elbows and lower yourself down to the ground as slowly as possible. You should try and take as many seconds as you can to go from the top of the movement to the bottom. Once you are as low as possible, simply drop off the dip bar. Do not worry about pushing yourself back up yet, as you will not be strong enough for that. Concentrate on performing slower and slower negatives, and over time, you will become much stronger. Eventually you will be able to perform the proper dip, having built much of your strength using the negative phase of the movement.

You should be aiming to perform 3 sets of 10 repetitions, but if this is not possible, simply start with as many as you can manage and then build from there.

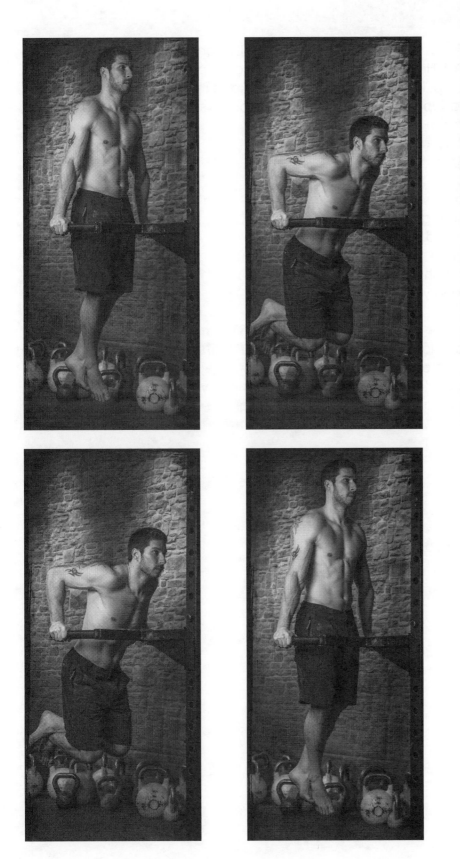
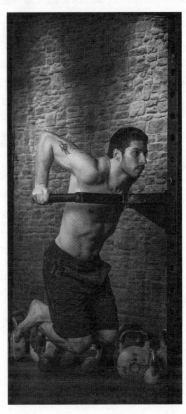

Front Dip

The front dip is one other triceps dips variation that we can look at. Here we use a single bar to perform the dip, instead of two parallel ones, and we adopt exactly the same hand position as seen in the top part of the muscle-up, which is an exercise we will look at in Chapter 8.

1. Stand with the bar in front of you and grab it with a shoulder width grip with your palms facing the ground.

2. From here either jump or push up until your elbows are straight and your body is resting against the bar.

3. Now bend your elbows and lower your body towards the bar. You may have to lean forwards and let your legs go forwards to help with the balance.

4. From the bottom position push back up until your arms are straight again. This counts as one repetition. You should try and perform 3 sets of 10 repetitions.

Teaching Points

For the front dip, you will want to progress in much the same way as for the triceps dip.

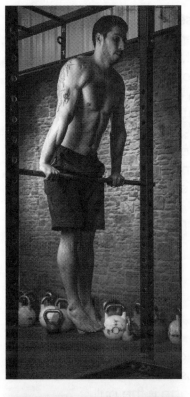
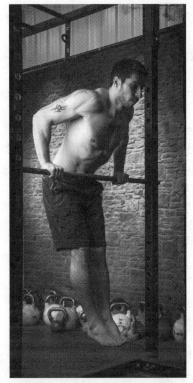
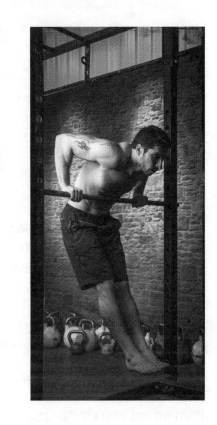

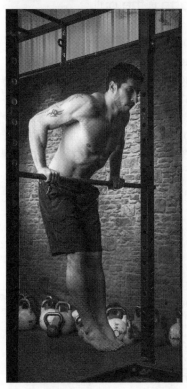
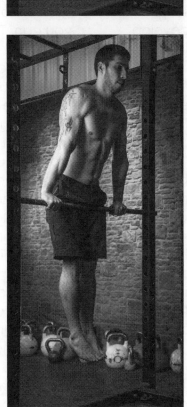

Once you are proficient in the pull-up variations presented so far, you can start to train towards the muscle-up. The muscle-up can be thought of as a combination of a pull-up and a triceps dip, and can be performed on either a pull-up bar or gymnastic rings. They can be performed at speed, which requires more of a powerful movement, or slowly, which requires a huge degree of strength and control. Within this section you will learn how to perform two different variations; the normal, or fast muscle-up, and the slow, or false grip muscle-up.

This exercise has seen a big increase in popularity in recent years, especially with the rise of CrossFit. However, I am not going to teach you any kipping muscle-ups here. Kipping is the technique used to basically cheat your way through the transition, which is the middle and most difficult part of the movement. If you kip or use momentum to move through the transition, then there is absolutely no point in performing the muscle-up at all. You may as well just do pull-ups and dips separately.

Normal Muscle-up

The normal muscle-up is where the majority of people begin with their muscle-up training, as you do not have to develop the false grip, which is required for the slow muscle-up. The road to actually getting your first muscle-up can be a long and difficult one, but once you achieve your first repetition you should be well on your way.

The muscle-up consists of three basic stages: the pull, the transition, and the push. The pull occurs from the bottom position to where your chin is over the bar. The transition is the stage where your shoulders go from a position underneath the bar to over it, and the push is where you straighten out your arms until you are above the pull-up bar at the top of a dip position.

1. Grasp the bar with an overhand grip with your hands about shoulder width apart. Swing forwards slightly, with straight arms.

2. As your body starts to swing back, pull yourself towards the bar as powerfully as you can. This stage is the pull.

3. As you reach the top of the movement, rotate your hands forwards so that your palms are facing back towards you. This movement must be quick and needs to happen with snap! You will need to loosen your grip on the pull-up bar slightly to allow your hands to rotate freely. This stage is the transition. This can be seen in the pictures that follow, where the shoulders move from underneath the bar to above it.

4. You should now be in the bottom position of a front dip (see page 158). From here, push up until your arms are straight. This stage is the push.

5. Reverse the movement until you reach the start position. This counts as one repetition.

Teaching Points

Even if you are proficient with all of the other pull-up variations, the muscle-up will probably cause you some trouble. Problems will usually arise in any one of the three stages of the movement, i.e. the pull, the transition, or the push.

To help strengthen the pull you should simply perform more pull-ups, but you should also concentrate on doing them as strongly and as powerfully as possible. Do a low number of repetitions, and concentrate on putting as much power and effort into each one as possible. You should be trying to get your chin as high above the bar as possible, as this will help when it comes to performing the transition stage. In addition, you can use weighted pull-up to increase your pull-up strength here; when you finally take off the added weight, the pull should feel much easier.

The transition is no doubt the most challenging part of the fast muscle-up, as it is the point at which the hands turn over, and the point at which the shoulders go from being below the bar to above it. To strengthen the transition there are a number of principles that you can apply:

- Firstly, when reaching the top of your pull-up, try to keep pulling, even if you do not move. This will engage all of the muscle groups that are responsible for the transition, and will allow strength to develop in that area.

- Secondly, you can use your legs to help with the pull to make the transition easier. To do this, simply raise your legs as you pull yourself towards the bar. In CrossFit circles this is known as "kipping", which simply means that we are using other body parts to help with a movement that does not involve those body parts

directly. As you become stronger, you must reduce the amount of kipping you use to make the exercise more challenging and build more strength.

- Lastly, if you lack the strength to push yourself up above the bar, then simply practice triceps dips and front dips until your strength in this area increases.

Keep practicing all of these different stages until you can put them all together and perform the muscle-up properly.

As the muscle-up is such a powerful movement and uses plenty of energy, you should start by trying to do 3 sets of 3 repetitions. As you become stronger and more efficient at the movement, try and increase this number.

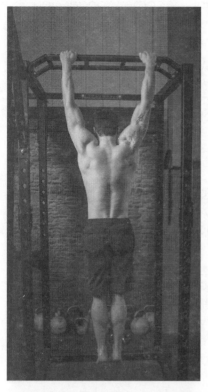

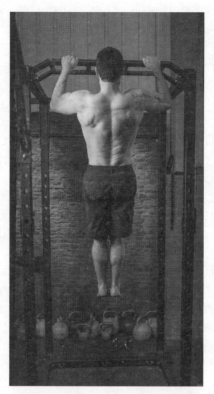

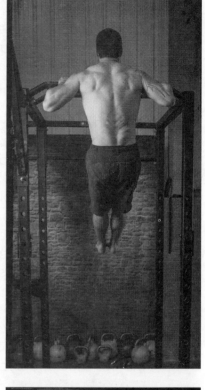

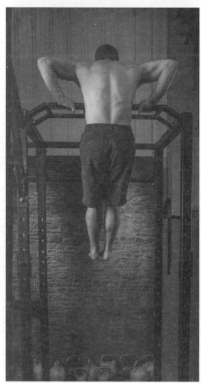

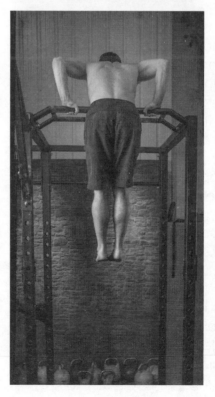

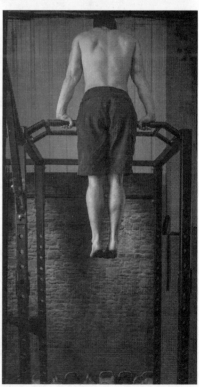

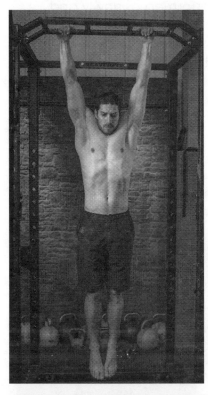

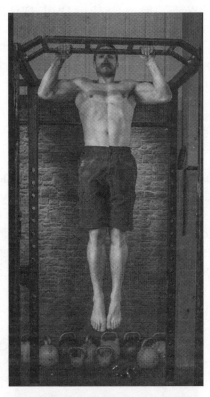

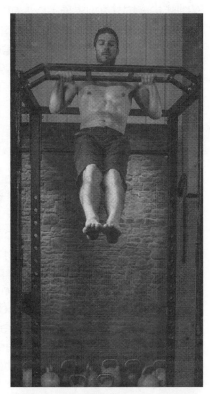

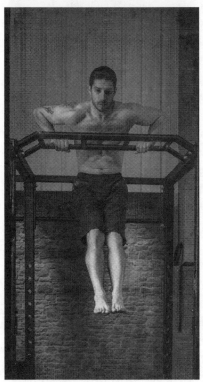

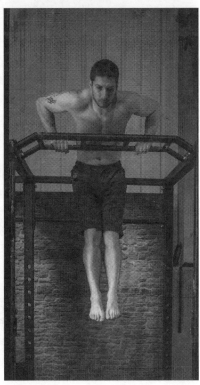

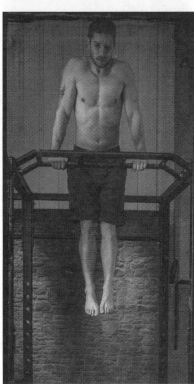

False Grip Muscle-up

Whilst the fast muscle-up is an awesome feat of strength and athleticism, the variation known as the false grip muscle-up is a display of pure, raw, controlled strength. Here, the pull, the transition, and

the push are performed as slowly and as strongly as possible, which makes the exercise much more challenging. This exercise should be your main goal when you start your muscle-up training.

Developing the False Grip

The first element to learn when attempting the muscle-up is a technique called the "false grip". This is simply a way of holding the pull-up bar that allows a greater degree of control, especially when combining pulling and pushing movements. The idea is not to grip the bar in a conventional way, but rather to position the wrist on top of the bar and curl the fingers round to rest on the back. This makes the top of the hand face the sky, which allows the slow transition from a pull into a push.

1. Place the heels of your hands on the top of the pull-up bar itself. I recommend placing some chalk not just on your palms, but also on your wrists, which will increase the friction generated and allow for a stronger grip.

2. Now wrap your fingers around the bar as best you can. Depending on the thickness of the bar and the size of your hands this will either enable you to place your fingertips behind the bar or on top of it. The top of your hands should now be facing the ceiling. If they are not, then readjust until they do.

3. Now attempt to hang using this grip. Most likely you will feel a huge stretch in the wrists and forearms, and probably a lot of cramping as well. This is normal,

and is just an indication of the lack of strength in your wrists and forearms. Also, locking out the elbow will be difficult when you first attempt this. Persevere and your flexibility will increase in time.

Teaching Points

At first you may not even be able to get into a false grip on a pull-up bar, and the action of hanging may be totally impossible. If this is the case then you should practice in the row position (see page 110). Simply hold this position for as long as you can, and as you become stronger, move onto the false grip on the pull-up bar.

Once you have built up some strength just hanging in the false grip, you should attempt some false grip pull-ups. These are simply pull-ups but with your hands in a false grip, and will get you used to pulling at the same time as performing the false grip, which is very difficult for most people.

In terms of the number of sets and repetitions you should perform, you should aim to hang for as long as you physically can, whilst keeping the false grip position. Aim for 5 to 6 sets of 10 seconds.

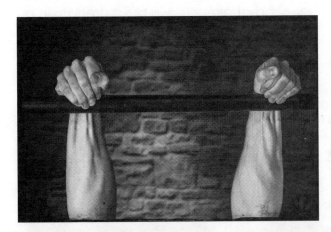
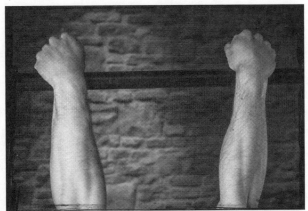
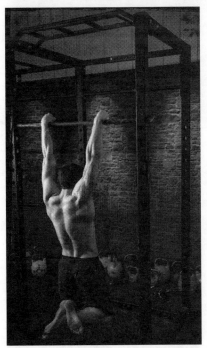
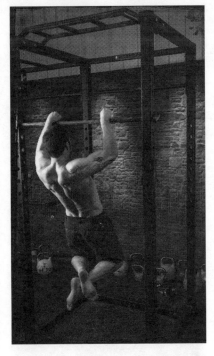
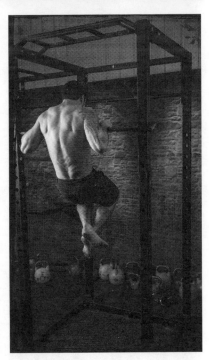

Working the Transition

The transition is easily the most difficult part of the muscle-up because it is a position in which it is very hard to exert force. There are two main methods we can use to build strength in the transition:

1. The first method is to pull yourself to the top of the pull-up and then try and pull up and over the bar. At first it will feel impossible, but gradually your strength will increase. The more time you spend in this position, the better you will become.

2. The second method is to start above the bar in the top position of the dip, and then to lower yourself down as slowly as possible. This method, also known as the negative phase and which we have looked at already, will build strength in a gradual way, and will enable you to work the movement without actually being able to do a false grip muscle-up.

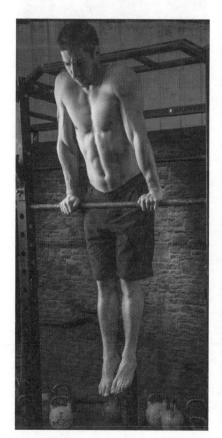 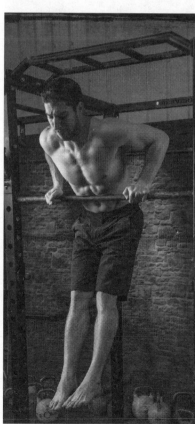 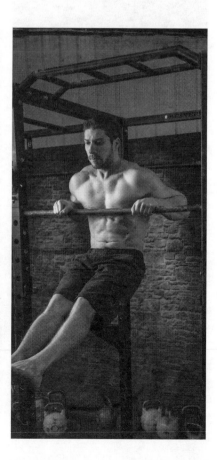

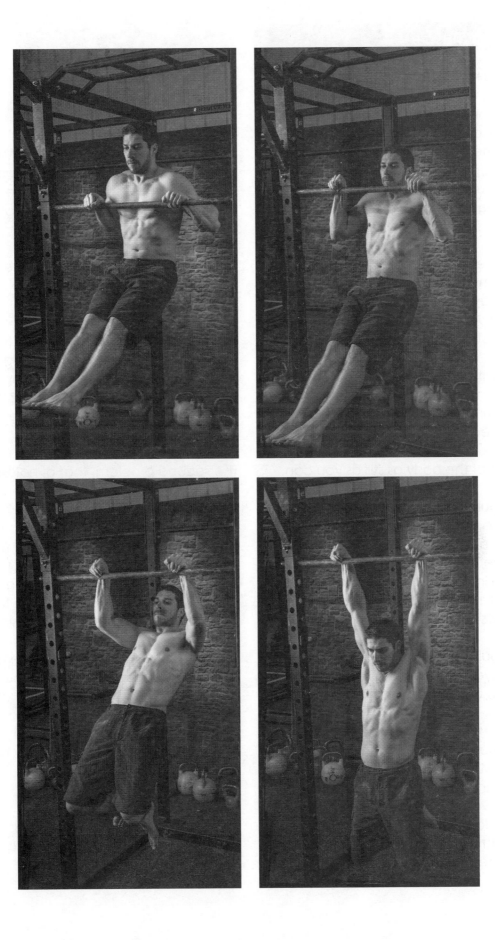

False Grip Muscle-up

Once you have spent enough time practicing the false grip, can hang in it for 30 seconds or so, and can perform a number of false grip pull-ups, it will be time to attempt a false grip muscle-up. The whole point of this exercise is strength and muscular control, so do not try and rush through it at any point. If you cannot perform it slowly, then it is not worth doing.

1. Grab the pull-up bar in a false grip with your hands about shoulder width apart. If you have it, make sure to apply chalk to both your palms and the undersides of your wrists.

2. Hang with completely straight arms, and then start to pull up slowly and strongly. Make sure to pull your scapulae down as described in the mobility section. Try not to use your legs to help you, and keep the rest of the body as still as you can.

3. Keep pulling strongly as your chin goes over the bar, aiming to transition into the push. It helps to slightly roll the shoulders over the hands at this point. Moving your legs up into an "L" position can help as the extra bodyweight in front of the bar can assist in rolling the shoulders forwards.

4. Keep pulling until your shoulders are above your hands. From here, simply push up until your arms are straight.

5. Then lower yourself down reversing the movement until you reach a dead hang again. Make sure that you keep the hands and wrists in the false grip position on the way down, as this will enable you to do multiple repetitions without constantly resetting your grip. This counts as one repetition.

Teaching Points

Even though it sounds relatively simple, the false grip muscle-up is one of the most challenging skills to master. There are two key points; the first is that you need to be able hold the awkward position of the false grip and pull at the same time, and the second is that you need to be able to move through the transition stage without using momentum or speed to help you.

The first problem, that of not being able to hold the false grip and pull at the same time, can be solved by practicing false grip pull-ups, as described on page 164, 'Developing the False Grip'. The strength built here will transfer directly over to the muscle-up.

The second problem, that of not being able to move through the transition slowly, can be fixed by performing slow negatives. To do this, get above the bar into the top position of the muscle-up by any means necessary. You can use a training partner to help you, a tall box to stand on, or any other suitable method. From this top position, lower yourself down as slowly as possible, particularly during the transition. You should be trying to reach the point at which the shoulders go from being above the hands to below them as slowly as possible. This will ensure that you hit all of the muscle groups involved in the movement. Simply repeat this for as long as necessary until you can perform the false grip muscle-up correctly.

In terms of sets and repetitions, as the false grip muscle-up is so demanding and should be performed slowly, you should aim to perform 3 or 4 sets of 2 to 5 repetitions.

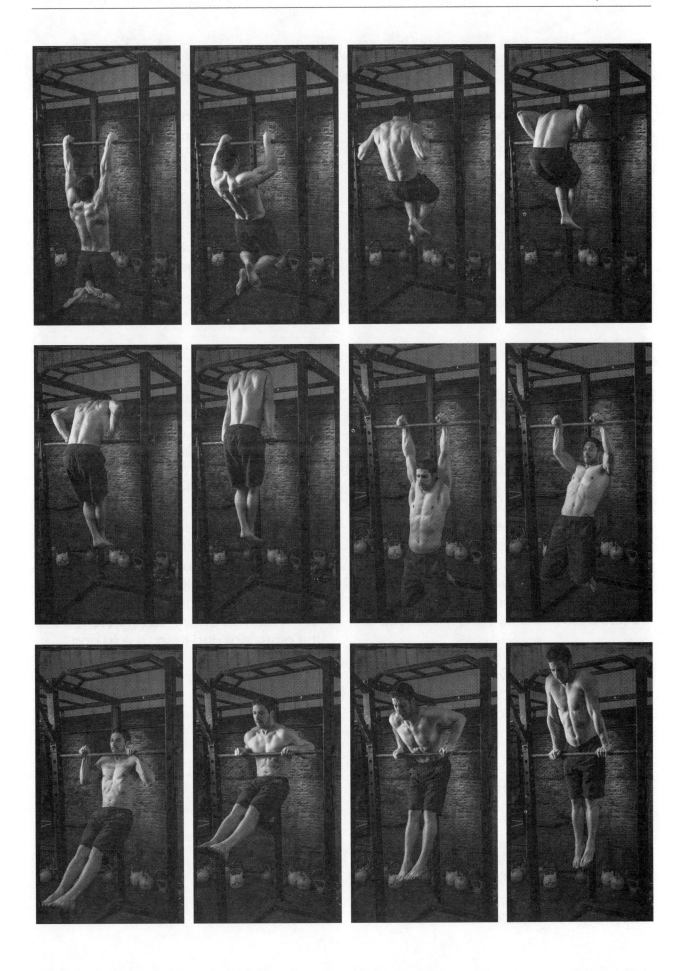

The third group of upper body pushing exercises is the handstands. Handstands literally place a demand on every muscle group in the body, from the hands, shoulders, back, and core, to lower body. Developing the handstand will be a major achievement in your calisthenic training. If you think about it, your legs are the strongest part of the body for the simple fact that they carry around your entire bodyweight all day, every day. Spending time in the handstand will develop the upper body in the same way that walking, squatting, lunging, and running does for the lower body.

We will look at all of the variations of the handstand in this chapter. The first task is to perfect the freestanding handstand. There are a number of stages to this and we will look at them next.

Wall Walks

If you have never attempted handstands before, then you may be very apprehensive about positioning your body upside down; in my experience this is the major stumbling block for the majority of people. To progress with the handstand group of exercises you must be completely confident when your body is inverted. To build this confidence we can use an exercise called wall walks. This movement will allow you to become more comfortable in the handstand position, and will also build real strength in the shoulders.

You will need to have a solid wall that will be able to bear your weight, and that has no obstacles to the front or side. It may also be a good idea to use mats to ensure you feel safe enough to progress with the exercise.

1. Place your feet at the bottom of the wall and get into the push-up position.

2. From here start to walk your feet up the wall. At the same time begin to move your hands back towards the wall. Take small steps and keep your arms and legs as straight as possible.

3. As you move up the wall keep your core as tight as you can, and do not allow your hips to drop towards the wall. Keep your head in a neutral position.

4. Walk your feet up the wall as far as you are able to. Begin by positioning the body at a 45-degree angle, and as you become stronger and more confident, move further and further up. Hold this position for a couple of seconds and then walk the hands forwards and legs down the wall again, taking care to keep the arms, legs and torso as rigid and straight as possible. You should be aiming to hold the position for 3 or 4 sets of 15 to 20 seconds.

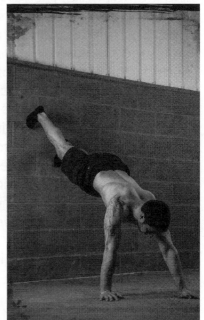

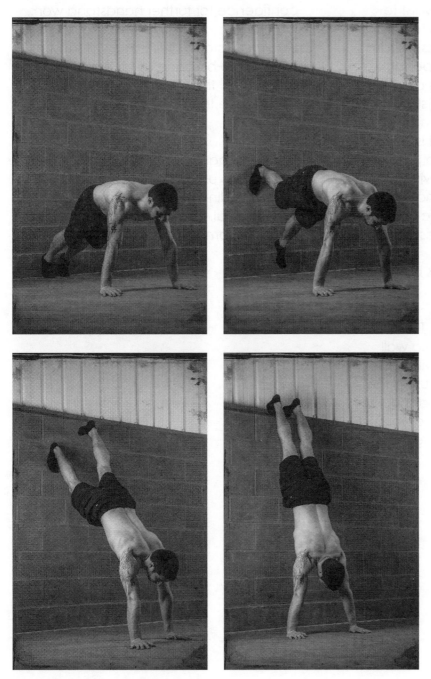

Learning How to Handstand

Once you have spent some time familiarising yourself with being inverted using the wall walks, you will want to start learning how to progress towards a freestanding handstand. This, as the name suggests, is where you perform a handstand with no support at all, using your fingers, hands, arms and shoulders to balance in one place. This is as much a strength exercise as it is a skill, so to progress you will need to practice regularly. Nevertheless, achieving a proper freestanding handstand is a vital component of your calisthenic training, and is well worth the time investment.

The freestanding handstand is best learnt in stages:

1. Wall-supported handstand. The hands are placed on the floor and a wall supports the feet, and this will teach you how to start balancing using the fingertips and the elbow and shoulder joints to control the rest of the body. It will also expose you to kicking up into a handstand in the first place.

2. Recovering from a handstand. This is a vital stage and is essential for building the confidence for further handstand work.

3. Floor handstand. This stage will show you how to balance using the fingertips, hands, and the elbows and shoulders to manipulate the body and maintain the handstand.

4. Parallette handstand. This stage will show you how to use parallettes to balance with, including using the apparatus to its full potential, and the pros and cons to using equipment for the handstand.

Wall-supported Handstand

The first stage in learning how to perform a freestanding handstand is the wall-supported variation. As the name suggests, this version allows the feet to rest on a wall so that you do not have to worry about tipping over. This is the most common concern for the majority of people when they start their handstand training, because going over onto your back makes you feel like you have lost control, and it can be very difficult to rebuild confidence if this does happen. If you overbalance onto your back, your feet will simply hit the wall and you can start again. Secondly, if you under balance onto your front, you can kick up into a wall-supported handstand and begin again.

The other main part to this exercise is that of kicking up into a handstand in the first place. This can be a problem for many people, but if you follow the instructions laid out below, you should not have too many difficulties.

This exercise is divided into two separate parts: **kicking up into the wall-supported handstand** (part 1) and **learning how to balance** (part 2).

Part I: Kicking up into the Wall-supported Handstand

1. Place your hands on the floor about a foot away from the wall you are using. The hands should be about shoulder width apart with the fingers spread out in a wide span.

2. Position your feet with one tucked up close to your chest, and the other stretched out behind you. Some people prefer to have the right foot forwards and the left foot back, and others prefer the opposite. Experiment with both to find which is your preference.

3. From here, kick up into the air with your rear leg. Try and keep it as straight as possible. Make sure that you keep your arms locked out and your core as tight as you can.

4. As your rear leg travels into the air, follow it with the front leg. At first, only kick up a small amount so that you can become comfortable with the movement. As you gain confidence, start to kick up harder and harder until your body becomes a little more vertical.

5. Once you become vertical, allow your legs to keep moving and they will hit the wall. This skill no doubt will be nerve-racking in the early stages, but keep persevering.

6. Once your feet are on the wall, hold the position for as long as possible. You should aim to perform 3 to 5 sets of 15 to 20 second holds.

7. Once you are ready to come down, keep the arms locked and allow one leg to drop before the other. Try to control the descent as much as possible, as this will also build strength and control.

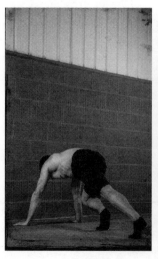
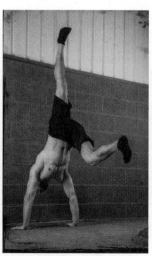
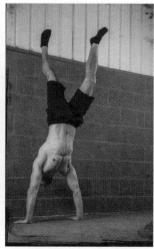
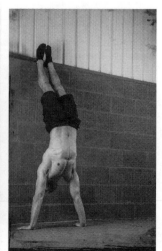

Part II: Learning How to Balance

The second part of the wall-supported handstand is learning how to balance. This is another very important component and must be practiced regularly to see improvement and progress. At first you will only be able to balance for a very short time, maybe a couple of seconds or so, but this will slowly improve and after a few weeks or months, you will be balancing for longer and longer periods.

1. Kick up into a wall-supported handstand and get comfortable.

2. From here, push down with your fingertips as hard as you possibly can. It helps to have the middle of the fingers slightly raised off the ground, as is shown in the right-hand picture. You should be aiming to get your feet to come away from the wall. If pushing down with your fingertips does not move your feet off the wall, try kicking very softly off the wall with your feet.

3. As soon as your feet come away from the wall balance for as long as you can. To correct overbalance (onto your back) push down hard with your fingertips. To correct under balance (down onto your front), bend your elbows slightly, and try and manipulate your shoulders. If at any point your feet hit the wall, then push back off and try again. If you under balance and land on your feet, then simply kick back up into a handstand again.

4. Practice for as long as you are able. When your shoulders and upper body become too fatigued, take a rest and then perform another set.

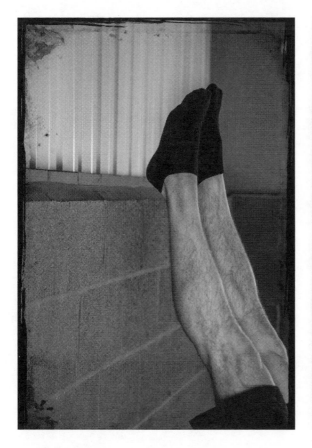
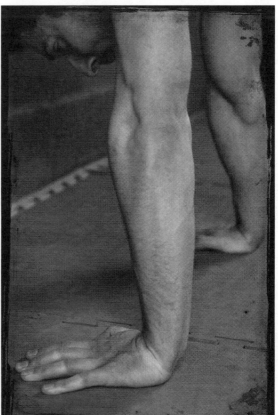

Recovering From A Handstand

Once you have built your confidence kicking up into a handstand and resting your feet against a wall, and you have generated some strength in the hands and fingers and can balance a little, then it is time to start trying to kick up into a handstand without a wall to catch you. This can be daunting at first as most people are scared of falling onto their backs and hurting themselves. To avoid this, and to give you more confidence, you need to learn how to recover from a handstand and make sure you practice this skill. This will give you much more confidence when it comes to actually performing freestanding handstands.

1. Find a clear space free of obstacles that you may hit or run into. Now kick up into a handstand.

2. As you feel your legs going over your head, as if you are going to overbalance, take one hand off the floor. You will probably have a preferred side for this. For example, I always take my left hand off the floor when recovering from a handstand.

3. Taking your hand off the floor will make your body pivot around the hand that is still in contact with the floor, and your legs should come round at the same time.

4. Then simply place your feet on the floor and recover from the handstand. Keep practicing until you are completely comfortable doing this. You need to be confident that you can recover every time you overbalance. Simply spend as much time as you need to perfect your recovery technique.

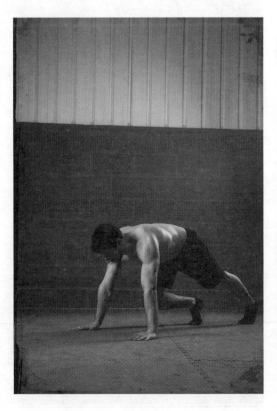
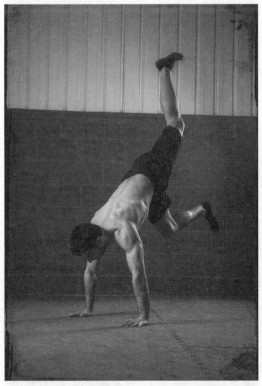

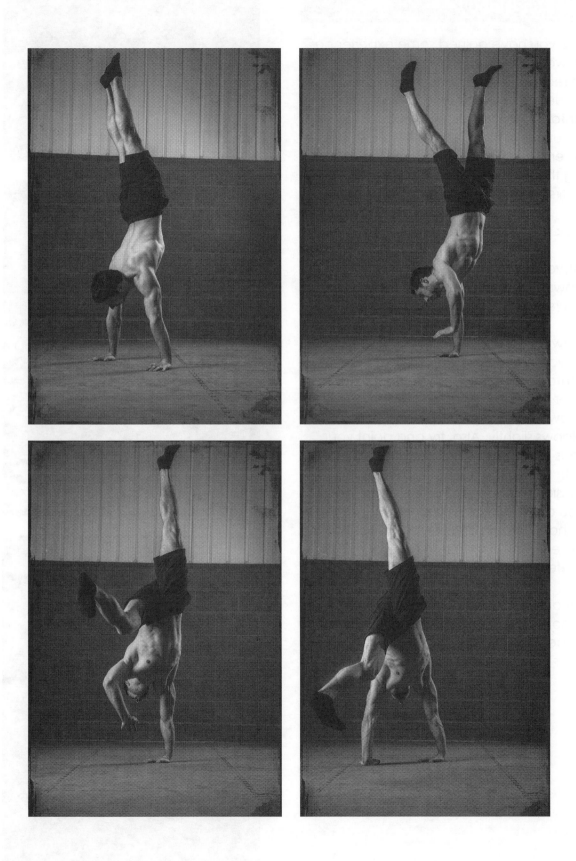

Floor Handstand

Once you have gained some experience with wall-supported handstands and can recover from a handstand with confidence, it will be time to start kicking up into a handstand and trying to balance without a wall for support. There are two different types of freestanding handstands: using the floor and using parallettes. We will look firstly at the floor handstand.

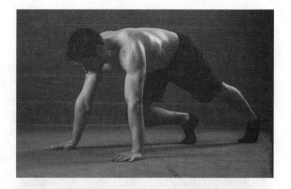

1. Kick up into a handstand.

2. As your legs come over your head, push down hard with your fingertips to stop yourself from overbalancing.

3. Now try and hold the handstand as long as you can. To correct overbalance (onto your back), push down hard with your fingertips. To correct under balance (down onto your front), bend your elbows slightly. Also, try and point your toes as much as possible, as this can help with both alignment and generating tension throughout the rest of the body. You can either press your legs together or hold them in a straddle "V" position. Experiment with both to find your preferred option.

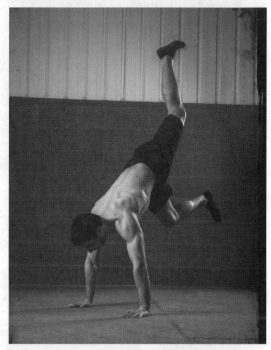

4. Try and hold the handstand for a set amount of time, such as 2 to 3 seconds to begin with. Slowly you will improve and your hold times will increase.

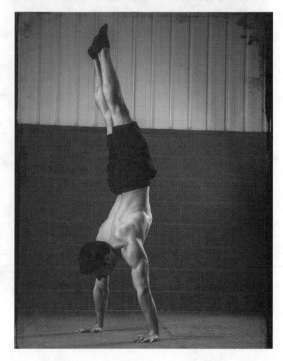

Parallette Handstand

The second type of freestanding handstand is performed on parallettes. I find this variation somewhat easier than when performed on the floor, as the use of the parallettes allows your hands to both pull and push, making balancing slightly easier in most cases. You will still need to practice to achieve proficiency though. There is also the added factor that parallettes will be a little higher, which means that when you recover you will be a little higher off the ground, which can be an issue for some people.

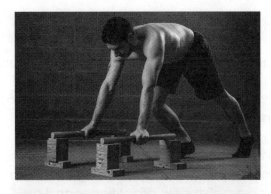

1. Position your parallettes about shoulder width apart and place your hands on them.

2. Kick up into a handstand. As your legs come over your head, push down hard with your hands to stop yourself from overbalancing.

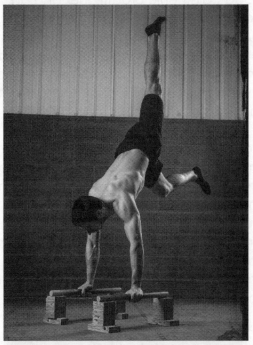

3. Now try and hold the handstand as long as you can. To correct overbalance (onto your back), push down hard with your hands. To correct under balance (down onto your front), pull hard with your hands and/or bend your elbows slightly. Also try and point your toes as much as possible, as this can help with alignment and generating tension throughout the rest of the body. You can either press your legs together or hold them in a straddle "V" position. Experiment with both to find your preferred option.

4. Try and hold the handstand for a set amount of time, such as 2 to 3 seconds initially. You will improve steadily and your hold times will increase.

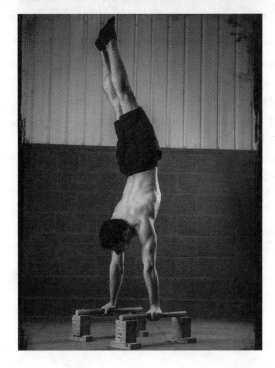

Handstand Push-ups

In addition to simply holding the handstand in a stationary position, we can also add a pressing or pushing action to create an even more challenging set of exercises, known as handstand push-ups. They combine strength, balance, and muscular control, and are the difference between a good calisthenic practitioner and an amazing one. You will probably find that your ability with the other exercises starts to improve after beginning your handstand training, and this is a common occurrence. In this chapter we will look at four different handstand push-ups:

1. Handstand push-ups with the hands on the floor and using the wall as a support.
2. Freestanding handstand push-ups with the hands on the floor.
3. Handstand push-ups with the hands on parallettes and using the wall as a support.
4. Freestanding handstand push-ups with the hands on parallettes.

1. Using the Floor with Wall Support

This variation is the starting point and the easiest of all of the handstand push-up exercises. As the name suggests, it is performed with the hands on the floor and the feet resting against the wall. This allows the head to only drop to the level of the hands, and you do not have to be able to perform a freestanding handstand either, as the feet are in contact with the wall.

1. Place your hands 8 to 12 inches away from the base of a sturdy wall.

2. Kick up into a handstand and allow your feet to carry over until they come to rest against the wall. Keep the core tight and the body as straight as you can.

3. From here, bend your elbows and allow your feet to slide down the wall. Keep going until your head nearly touches the ground. You can place a mat here if necessary.

4. Now push up hard until you reach the start position and your arms are straight again. This counts as one repetition.

Teaching Points

When starting handstand push-ups you may not have enough strength to push back up from the bottom of the movement. If this is the case, then we can use the negative phase of the exercise to help build enough strength to perform the exercise properly. To do this, kick up into a wall handstand. Then, bend your elbows and lower yourself down to the ground as slowly as possible. Try and make the descent take as long as your strength allows, trying to generate as much tension in the body as you can. Once your head reaches close to the ground, or your strength gives out, then allow your feet to come away from the wall and land on your feet. This counts as one repetition. From there, you would simply kick back up into a wall handstand again and repeat for the desired number of repetitions. Aim to do 3 to 4 sets of 5 repetitions to start with, and then increase the number as you become stronger.

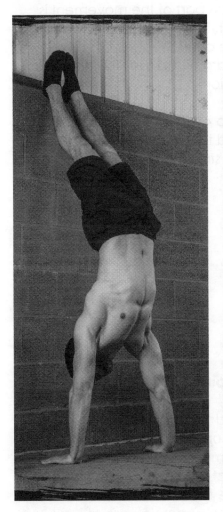
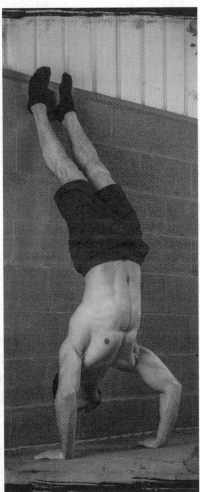
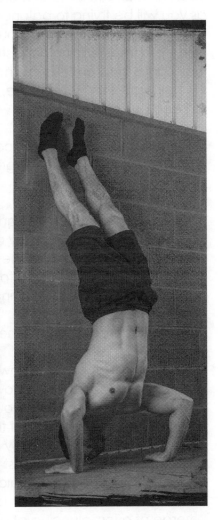

2. Using the Floor with No Support

After you have built some strength using supported handstand push-ups, it will be time to start trying to perform the same movement but without the wall to support you. This exercise is much more difficult as you will be trying to balance and exert strength at the same time. Your practice with both freestanding handstands and wall handstand push-ups with wall support will help you with this exercise, so make sure to keep performing them as well.

1. Place your hands on the floor, shoulder width apart. Splay your fingers out to aid with your balance.

2. Kick up into a handstand and allow your feet to carry over until they are vertical. Keep the core tight and the body as straight as you can. Get into a solid handstand before continuing. Your legs can either be in a straddle "V" position, or they can be held together.

3. From here, bend your elbows and allow your body to move towards the ground. Keep going until your head nearly touches the floor. At this point your body should be slightly angled and your elbows bent to at least 90 degrees. Constantly correct your balance as you descend. It is slightly easier to be on the verge of overbalancing at all times, as this will allow you to continuously exert some pressure through the fingertips.

4. Now push hard against the ground and straighten your arms until you reach the start position. Make sure to move the feet back over above the hands, otherwise you will either overbalance or under balance. This part of the movement is actually very difficult, as it is very easy here to lose control, especially if you push too hard or too fast. This counts as one repetition.

Aim to do 3 to 4 sets of 3 to 5 repetitions to start with, and then increase the number as you become stronger.

Teaching Points

Again, if you do not have enough strength to push back up, work with the negative phase of the movement until you do. Also, do not neglect working on building up your hold time for the normal freestanding handstand. The better you are at balancing, the easier handstand push-ups will become.

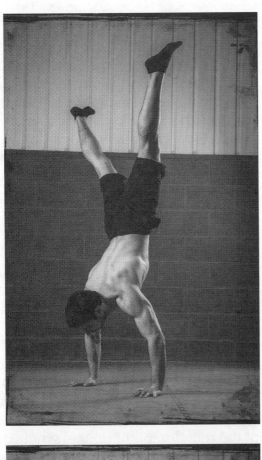

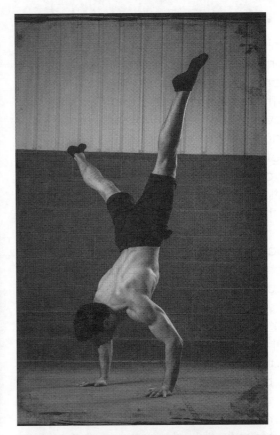

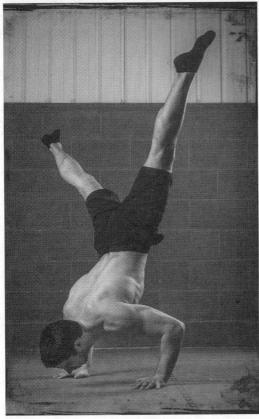

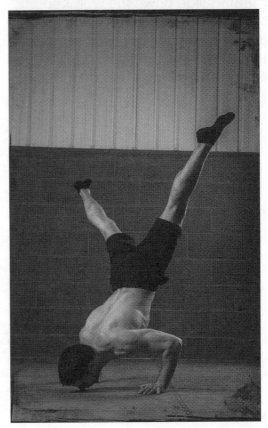

3. Using Parallettes with Wall Support

The third handstand push-up variation is performed on a set of parallettes or push-up bars with the feet supported on the wall. This allows the head to drop below the level of the hands, which increases the range of motion and allows greater strength to be built. It goes without saying that you should be proficient with the two variations presented so far before moving onto this version.

1. Place your hands on your parallettes, 8 to 12 inches away from the base of a sturdy wall.

2. Kick up into a handstand and allow your feet to carry over until they come to rest against the wall. Keep the core tight and the body as straight as you can.

3. From here, bend your elbows and allow your feet to slide down the wall. Keep going until your head nearly touches the ground. The aim is to get your hands level with the shoulders, but this will depend on your strength, flexibility, and the height of your parallettes.

4. Now push up hard until you reach the start position and your arms are straight again. This counts as one repetition. As this movement is more difficult than normal handstand push-ups, your repetition range will naturally be slightly lower. Aim to do 3 to 4 sets of 2 to 4 repetitions.

Teaching Points

As this variation uses a much wider range of motion, it is quite likely that you will struggle to push yourself up from the bottom position, especially when you first start training with them. As with the many other exercises that we have looked at so far, the best way of increasing strength using this exercise is to use the negative phase of the movement. To do this, simply get into the handstand, lower yourself down to the ground as slowly as possible, and then allow your feet to drop to the floor. Then repeat this for the desired number of repetitions.

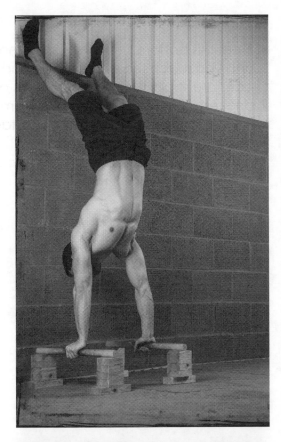
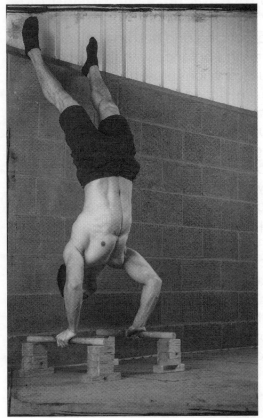
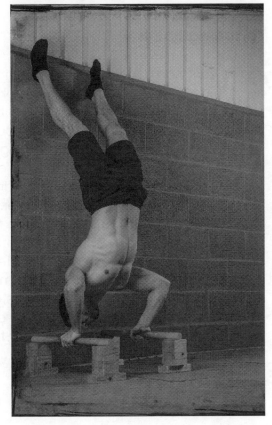
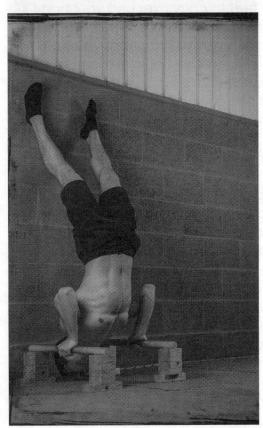

4. Using Parallettes with No Support

After practicing and building up your strength and balance with the handstand push-up variations presented so far, it will be time to work on the most difficult version; the free balancing handstand push-up with the hands on parallettes. Getting to this stage will be a major milestone in your upper body training, and once you can perform these you will find that your overhead pressing strength will be at a phenomenal level.

1. Place your hands on your parallettes and make sure they are stable and secure. Your parallettes should be about shoulder width apart, but set them up however is comfortable for you. Make sure that the area around you is free and clear of obstacles.

2. Kick up into a handstand and allow your feet to carry over until your body becomes vertical. Keep the core tight and the body as straight as you can. You can either have your legs together or in a straddle "V" position. Whichever body position you choose, make sure that the toes are pointed to help align the body.

3. From here, bend your elbows and allow your body to move towards the ground. Keep going until your head nearly touches the floor. The aim is to get your hands level with the shoulders, but this will depend on your strength, flexibility, and the height of your parallettes. As you descend you should allow your body to angle slightly. This is natural, and is a consequence of the way the shoulders are constructed, and the movement of your centre of gravity.

4. From this bottom position push up hard until you reach the start position and your arms are straight again. This counts as one repetition. Again, as this movement is more difficult than normal handstand push-ups, your repetition range will naturally be slightly lower. Aim to do 3 to 4 sets of 1 to 3 repetitions.

Teaching Points

As this variation is the most challenging of the handstand push-up variations looked at so far, it is very unlikely that you will be able to perform them perfectly on your first attempt. Initially, try reducing the range of motion to make them easier to handle. To do this, only lower yourself down as far as your strength will allow, and no further. As your strength builds you can increase the range of motion that you use, until your hands become level with your shoulders in the bottom position. In addition, the more time you spend balancing in a handstand, the more proficient you will become, and it will also make exerting strength whilst trying to balance much easier.

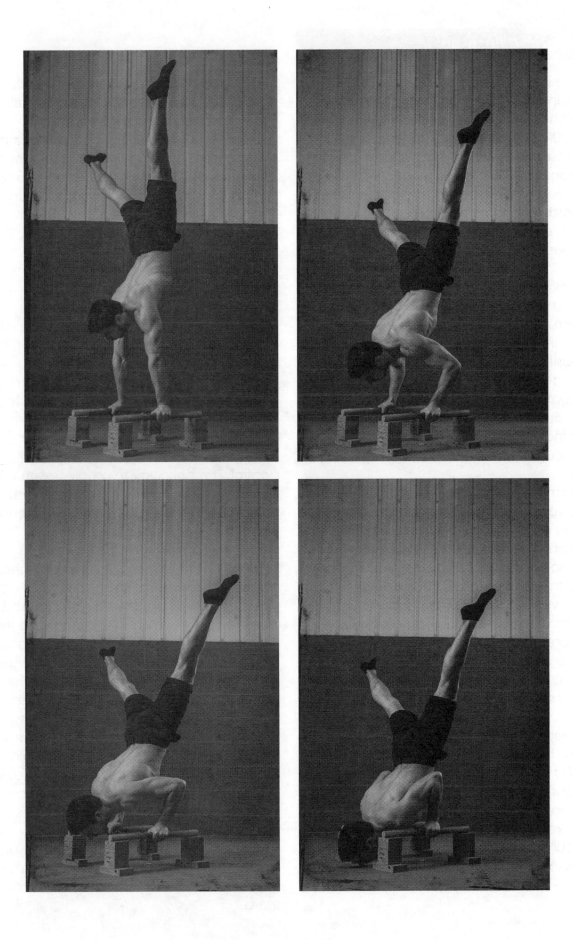

90-Degree Push-up

Once all of the handstand variations presented so far begin to become fairly straightforward, you can start to train for the 90-degree push-up. This exercise is a combination of a handstand push-up and a planche with bent arms, and will help to develop whole body muscular control and co-ordination. They are very difficult, but given enough time and training they should be possible for you to achieve.

1. Kick up into a freestanding handstand and get into a comfortable position. You can either use the ground or parallettes for this. Placing your legs into a straddle position (a wide "V" with pointed toes and locked knees) makes the movement slightly easier. Depending on your wrist flexibility you may need to turn your hands out slightly to allow the forearms enough freedom to move.

2. From here, start to bend the elbows and lower yourself down to the ground, as you would do in a normal handstand push-up. As you start to bend your elbows and your body starts to lower to the ground, allow your shoulders to move forwards of your hands. You should aim to make the body progressively more horizontal at the same rate as you descend. This will ensure that you maintain balance all the way through the movement.

4. Keep bending the elbows and levelling out the body until you reach the position of a planche with bent arms. This is when your entire body is horizontal, and your elbows are as bent as you can manage. To keep this position stable, try and press your upper arms into the sides of your torso, similar in principle to the elbow lever (see Chapter 10).

5. From this bottom position push back up hard, whilst reversing the orientation of your body so that it becomes progressively more vertical as your arms straighten. This stage will require a lot of control, as it is easy to either overbalance onto your back or under balance and land on your feet. Keep pushing up until you reach a handstand again. This counts as one repetition.

Teaching Points

This exercise will most likely give you a lot of trouble when you first start to train it, but this is completely normal. I know of no one that has performed this perfectly on their first attempt, so do not worry if it feels too difficult. The reason is that the 90-degree push-up demands extreme strength, extreme balance, as well as muscular control. The only way to progress with this movement is to keep practicing. The more you practice the stronger you will become, and so the easier the movement.

Working on movements like the planche, back lever, and all of the handstand variations will all contribute strength and athletic ability, which will in turn make the 90-degree push-up possible. Remember, with much of calisthenics there is a huge amount of carry-over from one exercise to the other, so if you feel that you are not progressing in one area, try moving your attention elsewhere and then come back to the exercise that you were having trouble with. The chances are that you will break through plateaus and sticking points more quickly and easily this way.

As for sets and repetitions, you will be lucky to get multiple repetitions — start with 2 to 3 sets of 1 repetition, and then build from there.

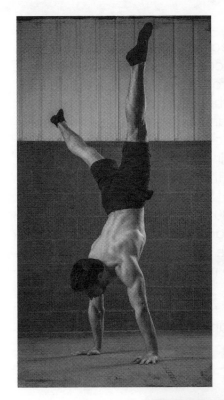
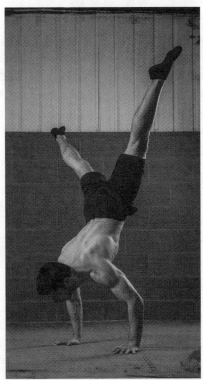
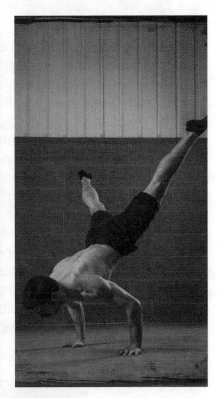
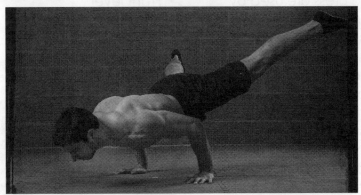
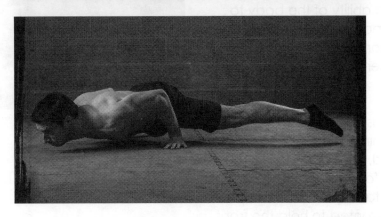

This next chapter contains all of the lever-type exercises. These are the planche, front lever, back lever, half lever, and human flag. Unlike the majority of the other exercises featured in this book, the levers are isometric exercises. Isometric simply means static, or unmoving, and requires you to hold a body position for a set period of time. This is different to a movement such as the pull-up, which has both a concentric phase (where you pull yourself towards the bar), and an eccentric phase (where you lower yourself down to the ground). Isometric exercises in general and the levers in particular are incredible for one major reason – building huge amounts of strength.

Just as the deadlift, back squat, bench press, and overhead press are used by strongmen to become hugely strong and powerful, the levers can be used by those that train using calisthenics to develop inhuman levels of strength, all without lifting a weight off the ground. This has to do with the way that all of the muscles contract when in a position such as the front lever. If we take the front lever as an example, we can see why it builds such huge strength. The force required to hold the position is extreme, but the ability of the body to exert force in this position is very small. This is the precise reason why the levers and the associated exercises are so good for building strength.

For all of the exercises in this chapter you will not be performing normal sets and repetitions. Instead, you will be trying to hold the positions for a set period of time, in as many sets as it takes you. For example, let's say that you wanted to hold the front lever for a total time of 30 seconds, but you could only hold the position for 3 seconds.

This would mean that you would perform 10 sets of 3 seconds to equal a total hold time of 30 seconds. As you progress do not increase the total hold time, but simply increase the amount of time you hold the position for in each set. For example, as your strength increases, you may do 5 sets of 6 seconds, then 3 sets of 10 seconds, then 2 sets of 15 seconds, and finally the total time of 30 seconds in 1 set. Once you hit this target and you are able to hold the position for the total time in one go, then it will be time to move onto the next stage of the exercise.

Within this chapter are the following movements:

- Planche
- Front lever
- Back lever
- Half lever
- Human flag

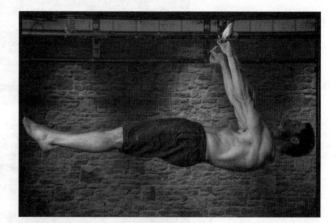

Planche

The planche can be thought of as the ultimate upper body pushing exercise. Like all of the exercises in this chapter, it is a static hold, and as such is designed to build unreal amounts of strength throughout the entire body. The planche is actually a graded gymnastics position, normally reserved for routines on the still rings or floor, and is used to demonstrate the gymnast's maximal strength. The essence of the planche is to hold the body horizontal, elbows locked out, with only the hands or fingertips touching the floor. At first glance the performer will seem to defy the laws of physics, but upon closer analysis the planche is simply a counter balance position. The weight of the upper body and the weight of the lower body will have to be evenly distributed for the planche to be successful.

In respect of the muscles being used, as the hands are the only part of the body in contact with the ground, the whole body must be tense otherwise the position will not be possible to maintain. The lower back, glutes, all of the muscles of the legs, and the entire core must contract with a huge degree of force to keep the torso stable. The upper body is also heavily taxed as well, especially the front of the shoulders, as they have to deal with the hugely decreased leverage because the lower body is so distant from the anchor point (the hands).

As with the other movements of this nature, the length of your limbs and your weight will have a very big impact on your ability to perform the exercise, as well as your rate of progress. Simply put, taller people, heavier people, and those with long limbs will find it more challenging to perform the exercises in this chapter. Do not be put off however; if you are a tall or heavy person you may well find these exercises very challenging, but the extra resistance will allow you to generate more strength than a shorter or lighter person. I have also personally seen very tall and heavy athletes performing the planche, so do not ever think that it is out of your reach.

There are a number of factors to achieving a true planche, not all of them immediately apparent, so we are going to look at a few of them. These are hand placement, supplementary exercises, and training time and volume for achieving the exercise.

Hand Placement

Hand placement can have a big effect on difficulty and comfort when training the planche, so below is a description of the different types of hand placement you can employ. Experiment with each one and see which is most suited to you. If you want (and I recommend that you do this), you can use all four hand positions to develop all-round planche ability.

- **Fingers facing forwards** – This method requires a great deal of wrist strength and flexibility, but does not place such a huge demand on the biceps as the other hand positions. This is the most common position for the majority of beginners, so it might make sense to begin here before trying other hand positions.

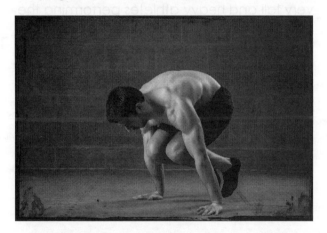

- **Fingers facing backwards** – This method requires huge strength from the biceps muscles, but does not require as much wrist flexibility. If you ever wish to graduate onto performing the planche on gymnastic rings, then this variation is essential. Most people find this hand position the most difficult out of all of them, simply because having the elbow open and exposed places a huge demand on the biceps and its associated tendons. This does have the added advantage though of building huge and extremely strong biceps, which is one of the reasons that so many male gymnasts have big arms.

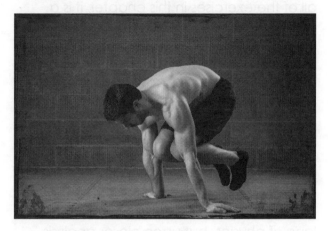

- **Using parallettes** – Using parallettes to perform the planche exercises is perhaps the most comfortable; the wrists are not taxed as much and you will have a greater deal of control over your balance. The disadvantage is that because the wrists are in a side on position, the forearms can be under a huge amount of stress. In my own experience with the planche, this caused me to have forearm splints for a time, where a shooting pain would rise up in the outer forearm. In retrospect this was probably because I had overtrained, and not through any particular use of parallettes for performing the planche.

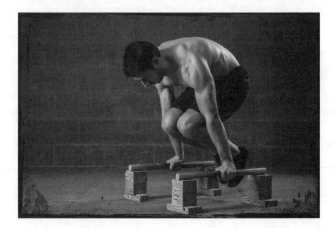

- **Using fingertips** – The last method is for those of you looking for even more of a challenge. Using the fingertips for the planche does not require much wrist flexibility, but will develop massive hand and finger strength, plus, if you pull one of these out of the bag next time you're at the gym, people will notice! The correct way to position yourself on your fingertips is to try and put the majority of the stress through the thumb joint, with the other fingers assisting and supporting. Needless to say, it can take a while to increase strength in the hands and fingers, so take your time with it and progress only at a rate that is sensible.

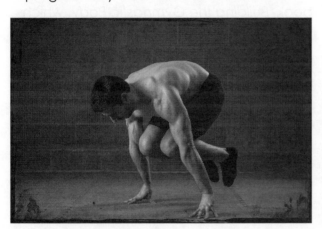

Supplementary Exercises

In addition to the actual planche exercises, like the tuck planche, straddle planche, etc., there are a number of supplemental exercises that need to be performed in conjunction with the planche exercises. Failure to perform these exercises is, in my opinion, the main reason why many fail to progress with the planche. The back lever, looked at later in this chapter, is one of these supplemental movements. On the face of it, the back lever does not look like it will help with the planche, but a closer look reveals why it is so important. The back lever develops the muscles of the lower back and core, as well as the glutes and

lower body, and more specifically, the ability of those muscles to hold the body in a horizontal position. This is exactly what the back, core, and lower body muscles are required to do in the planche, so training the back lever will obviously help to strengthen and progress your planche.

The other movements that help with the planche are the core exercises (such as the half lever) as these build huge core strength which is needed for all of the more advanced calisthenic exercises, and any of the movements that build straight-arm and shoulder strength and stability. It is worth looking at these exercises and making sure that they are a part of your routine, especially if your planche progress has slowed down or plateaued.

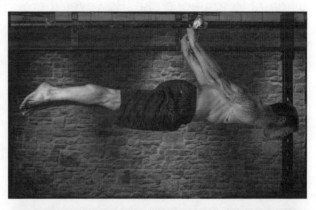

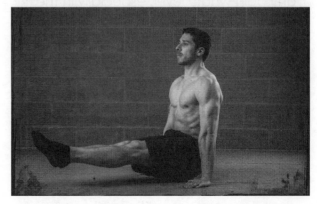

Training Time and Volume

Training the planche is not like training other movements, and is similar in principle to the other very demanding exercises such as the front and back levers, handstand push-up, one-arm pull-up, and hamstring curls. This is because it places huge demands on all aspects of the body including the muscles, tendons, and connective tissues. Therefore, it can take a while to recover from a workout where the planche was trained heavily. Knowing how often to train the planche and in what volume is one of the most common questions that I get asked. The answer is that this will be unique to everyone, as your genetics, training history, resilience to stress, diet, and recovery speed will be totally different to someone else. However, there are some points to bear in mind:

- Firstly, because the planche is such an intense exercise, initially you may want to limit your planche training to a maximum of 2 or 3 times a week at the most. This will give your body plenty of rest and time to recover before the next session.

- Secondly, if you start to experience any pain whatsoever, especially in the outside of the forearm (imagine a line drawn from your little finger to your elbow; the pain normally appears here if anywhere), then reduce the volume of your training immediately. I didn't do this and suffered for a long time with pain in the forearms when training the planche.

- Thirdly, listen to your body! Your body will tell you if it can handle extra training days or another repetition or two, and if it tells you that it is time to rest, it probably is.

Sets, Repetitions and Hold Times

When it comes to actually performing the planche exercises, normal sets and repetition ranges do not really apply. This is because the planche is a static exercise, and physically cannot be performed for repetitions in the traditional sense. In the case of the planche (and the half, back, and front levers), it is performed for a set amount of time that is decided before you start your workout. Ideally you want to build up slowly and increase your hold times until you can hold each position for a total of 30 seconds continuously. I first came across this idea in Coach Christopher Sommer's book, *Building the Gymnastic Body*, which lays out many beginning and fundamental gymnastic conditioning exercises. In it, Coach Sommer describes how to progress with static or isometric exercises in the following way; firstly, hold each position perfectly for a set amount of time (in our case 30 seconds) in as many sets as it takes you. For example, let's say my maximal hold time for the tuck planche is 5 seconds. This would mean that I would perform 6 sets of those 5-second holds to equal a total of 30 seconds. As you improve and become stronger, this would reduce to 3 sets of 10 seconds, and then 2 sets of 15 seconds and, finally, you will become strong enough to perform the 30-second hold continuously. Once you can do this then you would move onto the next stage in learning the exercise. Keep doing this until you reach the stage that you are aiming for.

Planche Lean

Although the planche lean is not an actual planche exercise, it is nevertheless the best entry point to planche training, as it will expose you to a number of factors that are common to the planche. These are; straight-arm strength, rounded shoulders with protracted scapula/shoulder blades, and a similar body position.

1. To perform the planche lean, get into a push-up position. You can use any of the four hand positions described on pages 192 and 193. Experiment to find the most comfortable for you.

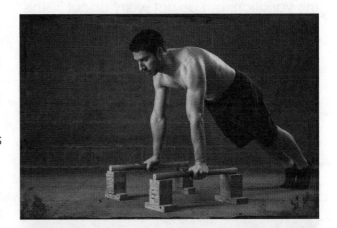

2. From this position, start to walk your feet forwards so your shoulders move forwards of your hands. Keep your elbow joints locked completely as you do this. If they start to bend, try and straighten them again or move your feet back slightly to make the movement easier.

3. From here push your spine up as high as possible, and separate your scapulae. Think about getting your shoulders to touch in front of you to make this happen.

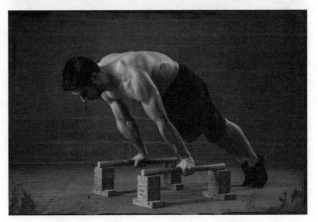

4. Get to the point at which you can only hold the position for 10 to 15 seconds and then hold. This counts as one set. Try and repeat for 3 to 4 sets.

Frog Stand

Once you have spent some time doing planche leans then you can begin supporting yourself on your hands using an exercise called a frog stand. The frog stand is an exercise popular in yoga, and will familiarise you with supporting your entire bodyweight on your hands.

Your elbows will have to be slightly bent for this variation, but do not worry about it. This is just because the legs have to rest on the arms. For all other exercises in this chapter, the arms must stay locked out.

1. Place your hands on the floor in front of you, fingers facing forwards or slightly out to the side, shoulder width apart. You can use any of the four hand positions described on pages 192 and 193. Experiment to find the most comfortable for you.

2. Place your knees on the outside of your elbows, as far forwards as you can manage. Your flexibility may be an issue here but this will improve with time.

3. Press down hard and lift your feet off the floor. You may have to lean forwards to balance, and there is a risk of falling onto your face. Having a soft mat in front helps here. Once you are balanced, hold the position for as long as possible.

Teaching Points

If you struggle to support your weight on your hands, then keep your feet on the floor at first. Gradually transfer more of your weight forwards onto your hands as your strength increases. If you find that this exercise hurts your wrists, try turning your hands out at an angle. This should serve to reduce the stress on them. As mentioned in the introduction to this group of exercises, you should aim to hold the position for 30 seconds in as many sets as it takes you, until you can hold the position for 30 seconds continuously. Once you can do this, move onto the next stage.

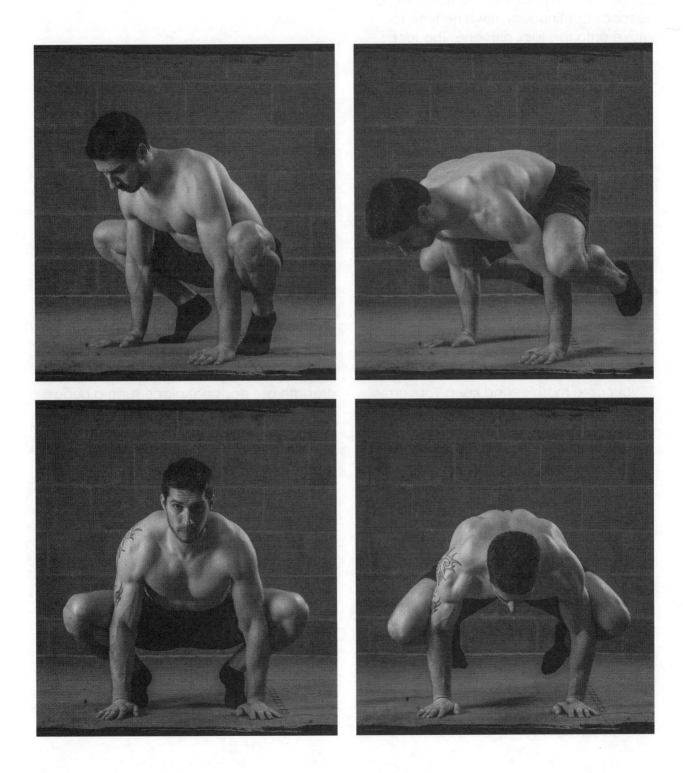

Tuck Planche

Once you can hold the frog stand for 30 seconds continuously, it will be time to move onto the tuck planche. The tuck planche is the first variation where you will be supporting your entire bodyweight using just your upper body, with completely locked elbows. This is an extension of the frog stand and requires a lot of arm, shoulder, and core strength. It is also the only variation from now on where a rounded back is allowed.

1. Place your hands on the floor, shoulder width apart, and position your feet together between them. You can use any of the four hand positions described on pages 192 and 193. Experiment to find the most comfortable for you.

2. Push down hard and lift your feet up. Tuck your knees into your chest using your core muscles and keep your arms completely straight. Do not allow your elbows to bend at all. Do not worry if the back is rounded, as this is straightened out in the next stage. Push your spine up and attempt to separate your scapulae. This is the hollow body position talked about in the planche lean.

3. Now hold this position for as long as possible.

Teaching Points

Moving from the frog stand to the tuck planche can be very difficult for the majority of people but there are a number of ways to make it a little more manageable. If you struggle to raise your feet off the floor you can use two raised objects each side of you to allow your feet to hang below the level of your hands; chairs, aerobic steps, or parallettes are suitable. This method allows you to build up the necessary wrist, arm, and shoulder strength but does not place such a huge demand on the core. As you become stronger, strive to raise the hips up until the feet and knees are higher than the hands.

As before, build up your hold time for a total of 30 seconds, in as many sets as it takes you. Keep working like this until you can hold the position for 30 seconds continuously. Once you can, move onto the flat back planche.

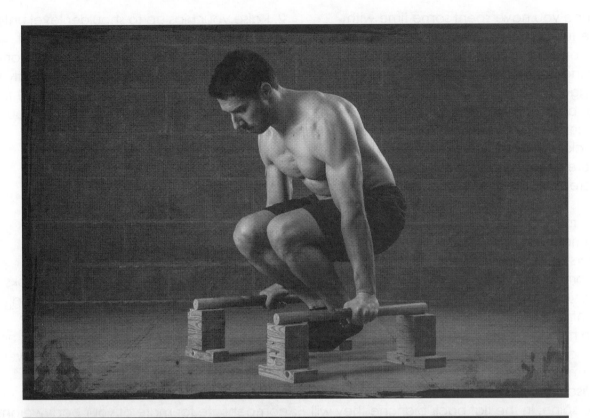

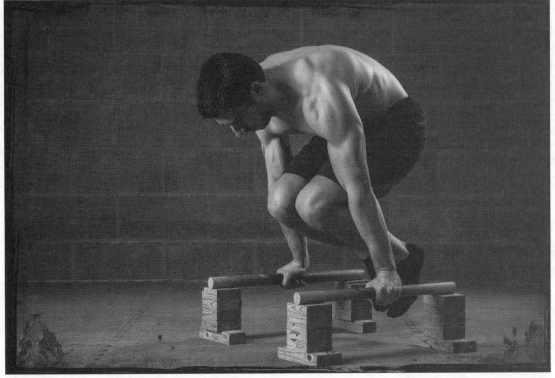

Flat Back Planche

Once you have spent some time with the tuck planche and can hold it for 30 seconds continuously, it is time to look at the flat back planche. As the name suggests, this variation is performed with a flat back. It is identical to the tuck planche, except that the hips are raised up and the back kept completely flat, which moves more of your bodyweight backwards, increasing the demand placed on the arms and shoulders. It also lengthens the front of the core, putting more of a demand on the torso. Even though it only looks like a small adjustment, you will be surprised at how much more challenging this variation is. It also forces you to control opposing muscle groups, namely the muscles of the abdominals and the muscles of the middle and lower back. In normal movement, these two opposing muscle groups act to either flex or extend the spine. In the flat back planche they will both have to contract against each other, whilst striving to hold a stable position. It can take quite a while to educate your body to behave like this, but keep practicing and it will come.

1. Get in the tuck planche position. You can use any of the four hand positions described on pages 192 and 193. Experiment to find the most comfortable for you.

2. Raise your hips up to shoulder level until you achieve a flat back. Think about tilting your pelvis forwards to do this, and you may have to lean forwards slightly to balance. Again, completely lock out the elbows. Push your spine up so that you reach the hollow body position.

3. Now hold this position for as long as possible.

Teaching Points

Even though the flat back variation looks very similar to the tuck planche, moving the hips up and back greatly increases the difficulty. This is because your back has to support the entire weight of your lower body, the front of your core is extended, and you have to lean forwards to compensate for more of your bodyweight being moved backwards. If you struggle to hold the position for any period of time at all, hold the tuck planche, raise your hips up momentarily, then lower them back down again. To allow steady progression we can use the same method as before. Build up to 30 seconds total time in as many sets as it takes you. Then keep working until you can hold the position for 30 seconds continuously.

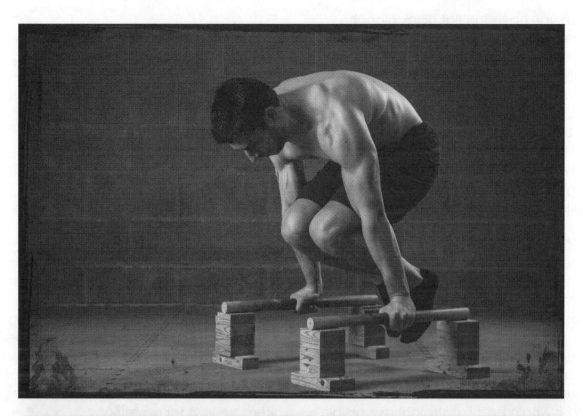

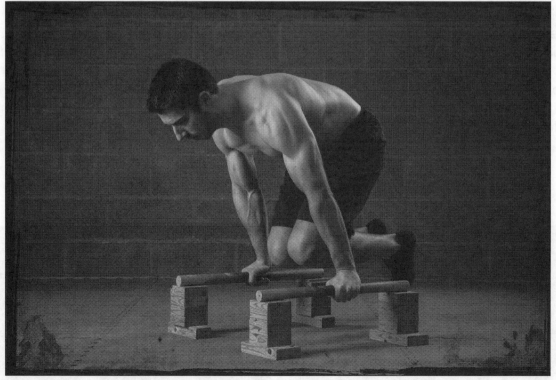

Single-Leg Planche

Once you have the flat back planche honed, and can hold it for 30 seconds continuously, then you can start to work on the single-leg planche. This stage is not quite as difficult as you may expect, because whilst one leg is stretched out to the back, the other leg is tucked up nice and tight underneath the core, which allows you to keep a large amount of your bodyweight close to your centre of gravity, making the movement easier.

1. Get into a flat back planche. You can use any of the four hand positions described on pages 192 and 193. Experiment to find the most comfortable for you.

2. Keeping one knee tucked tight into your chest, slowly extend the other leg out straight behind you. Strive to get your whole body as straight as possible. Pointing your toes as well will help to align the body. Make sure to keep the hollow body position as much as possible.

3. Hold this position. Make sure you work with each leg extended to work each side of your body equally.

Teaching Points

If straightening your leg out and holding it there is too challenging, then straighten it and immediately bring it back in again. Repeat this, trying to hold the leg out for longer periods every time. You can also alternate legs for repetitions.

Once you get to this variation do not worry about trying to hold the position for 30 seconds continuously. As it is such an intense movement, aim to hold it for a solid 20 seconds before moving to the next stage.

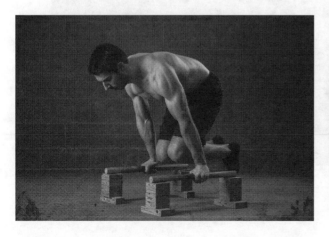

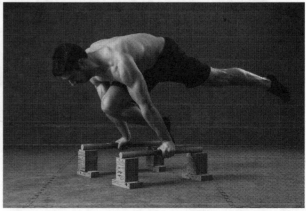

Straddle Planche

After you have become proficient with the single-leg planche, you can begin working on the straddle planche. As the name implies, this is performed with the legs in a straddle, or a "V" position. It goes without saying that the wider the straddle, the easier the exercise will be. This is because more of your bodyweight will be closer to your centre of gravity, making the lever shorter, requiring less strength to perform. Achieving the straddle planche will be a major breakthrough and many people stop here, not even bothering to learn the full planche. Whichever choice you make, know that the straddle planche is one of the most challenging calisthenic movements to perform, so do not be disappointed if it takes you a long time to master. The mistake most people make is thinking that it simply involves leaning far enough forwards so that the legs come off the floor. This is only half the story however, as the lower back, glutes, and core have to be strong enough to support the lower body. To overcome this problem, you should contract all of your muscles as hard as possible. If any part of the body is not under tension when you attempt these exercises, then you will not be able to perform them.

There are a number of ways of getting into a straddle planche:

1. From a tuck planche
2. Forward pull
3. Kick throughs
4. From a handstand

I have used all of the methods that I am going to describe at some point along my journey to get the planche, so it is well worth you experimenting with each of them until you find the one that is most beneficial to you.

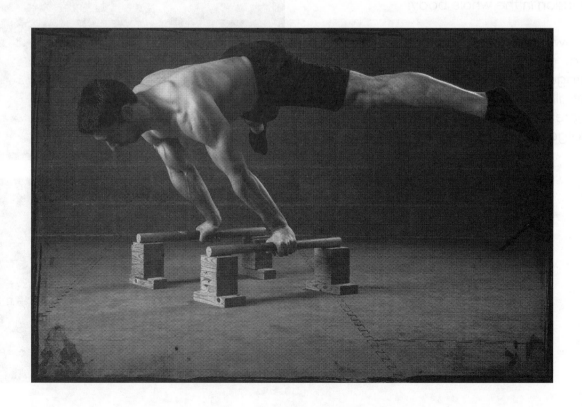

1. From a Tuck Planche

The first method of learning the straddle planche is moving from a simpler variation of the movement to the more difficult one. In this instance we will use the tuck planche and then move the legs out until we reach the straddle position.

1. Get into the tuck planche position. You can use any of the four hand positions described on pages 192 and 193. Experiment to find the most comfortable for you.

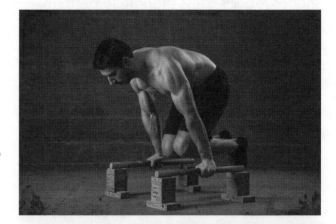

2. From the tuck position, slowly extend both legs in a wide straddle until they are straight behind you. You will have to lean forwards as you do this, and much of the success of the movement will be down to your ability to balance.

3. Strive to get your whole body as straight as possible. Pointing your toes will help to align the body. Contract all of your muscles as hard as you can to generate tension in the whole body.

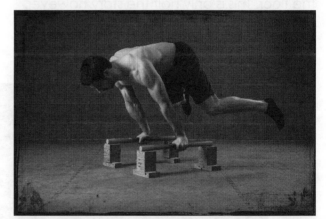

4. Now hold this position for as long as you can. As this is the penultimate stage to the planche, it is therefore very challenging. A hold time of 10 seconds here is very impressive, so this is a good target as you progress.

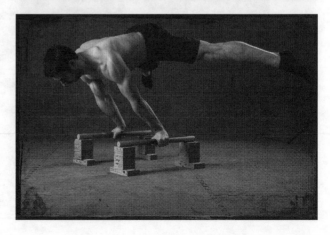

2. Forward Pull

The second method of learning the straddle planche is moving into it from a push-up position. This has many benefits, most notably the gradual nature of the transition.

1. Get into a push-up position with your legs in a very wide straddle. You can use any of the four hand positions described on pages 192 and 193. Experiment to find the most comfortable for you.

2. From here, start to lean forwards and "pull" your legs with you. Making the pull slow will enable you to gauge the balance needed much more accurately.

3. Keep a hollow body position and keep leaning forwards until your feet start to drift off the ground. It is fine here if your torso rises and becomes flat first. If this happens, then after your torso is in the correct position, contract your glutes and lower back hard to raise the legs up to the same level as the torso.

4. Once you reach the straddle planche position, hold it for as long as you can.

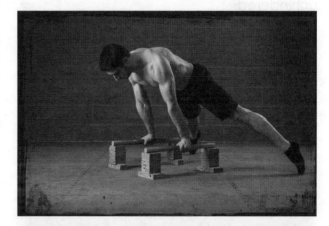

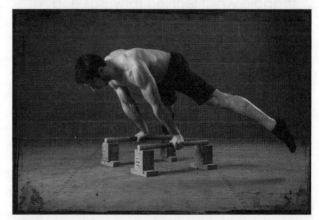

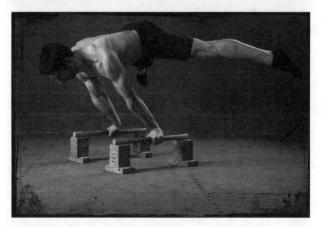

3. Kick Throughs

The third method of learning the straddle planche is using what I call kick throughs. Kick throughs allow you to use momentum and speed to get into the correct position for a split second before retracting your legs again. Kick throughs can only really be performed using parallettes, as you will need the extra height to allow the lower body to move between the arms unhindered.

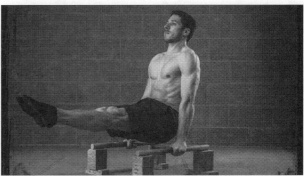

1. Place your hands on your parallettes and get into a half lever or a tuck half lever position. (If you are unsure of how to perform the half lever, turn to page 227 to see how.)

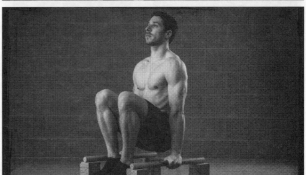

2. From here, move your legs through the gap in your arms and out to the back as fast as you can. In effect you will be trying to "kick" your legs into a wide straddle whilst leaning forwards and generating plenty of tension in the upper body and core.

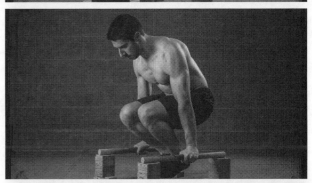

3. As soon as you reach the straddle planche position, hold it for as long as you can. At first this may only be a split second. Once you cannot hold it any longer, allow your legs to drop and come back through the gap between your arms again and resume the half lever position. This allows your shoulders to have a small rest.

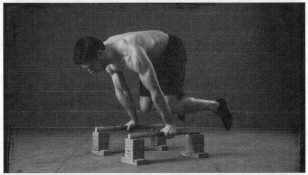

4. Repeat the kick throughs for as long as you can whilst maintaining good form.

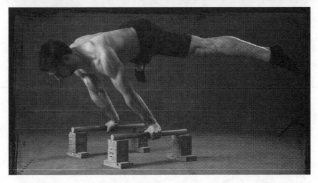

4. From a Handstand

The last and probably most difficult method of getting into the straddle planche is lowering into it from a handstand. Even though this sounds very difficult, it actually has a number of benefits.

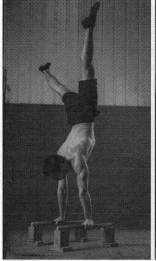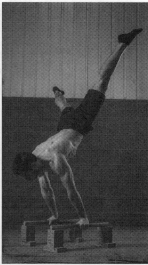

- Firstly, you can make the transition as slow as you want, allowing you to keep control over every aspect of the movement.

- Secondly, the descent acts as a slow negative, which will help build strength in exactly the same way as the other negative movements elsewhere in this book.

- Thirdly, it looks insanely cool, which is always a good reason for doing an exercise.

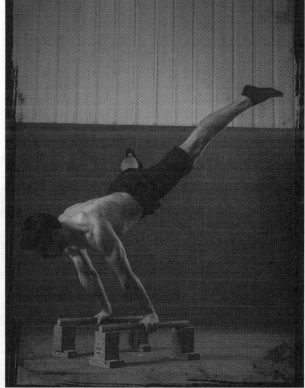

1. Get into a freestanding handstand. The hand placement you use for this is entirely up to you, but I prefer using parallettes as these afford a greater degree of control. Once you are in the handstand, place your legs in the widest straddle that you can.

2. From the handstand start to move the shoulders forwards whilst allowing the legs to drop. This is similar to the 90-degree push-up in Chapter 9 (see page 186), but in this case the arms have to remain completely straight.

3. Keep allowing the shoulders to move forwards and lowering the legs, until the whole body is horizontal and you reach the straddle planche position.

4. Now hold this for as long as you can.

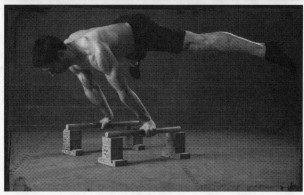

Full Planche

After putting in months of consistent work, you should be ready to attempt the full planche. This is essentially a straddle planche but where the legs are brought together. This small adjustment may take many weeks or months to perfect, as the leverage is decreased even further than with the straddle planche. When getting to this stage, even a 5-second hold is extremely impressive.

1. Position yourself in a straddle planche. You can use any of the four hand positions described on pages 192 and 193. Experiment to find the most comfortable for you.

2. There are two main ways you can move into the full planche. (1) Get into a straddle planche using any of the four methods described on pages 204–207. Then simply bring your legs together from the straddle position.

3. (2) Use any of the four methods described on pages 204–207 but start with the legs together.

4. Now hold this position for as long as possible. A 5-second hold is extremely impressive here, so do not worry if you struggle to hold for longer.

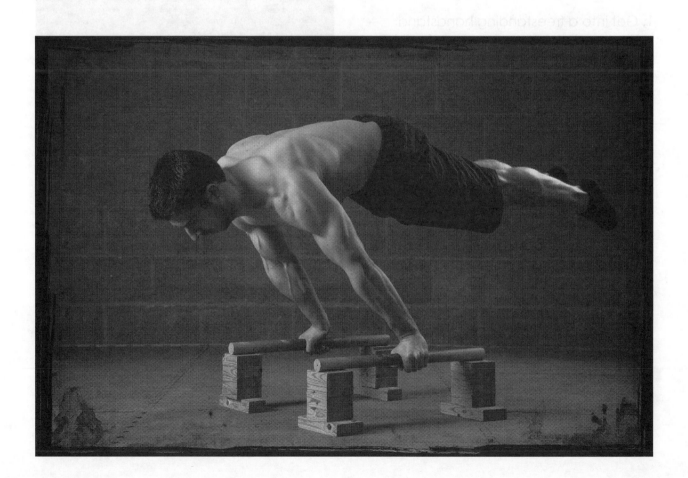

Planche Push-up

Although holding each position of the planche is an amazing individual exercise, we can add movement to this traditionally static exercise to incorporate even more variation and strength benefits. These come in the form of planche push-ups. Planche push-ups can be performed using each of the different variants, but obviously the more challenging the planche exercise, the more challenging the push-up will be.

1. Get into the planche variation of your choice. The pictures below show both a tuck planche and a straddle planche push-up.

2. From the top position, bend your elbows and start to lower yourself down towards the ground. Make sure that you keep the body position as perfect as possible.

3. Once you have gone as low as you are able to, push back up hard until your elbows lock out again. This counts as one repetition. Repetition ranges should be kept low, as you should be on the limit of your strength. For the more advanced variations, try and do 3 sets of 3 to 5 repetitions.

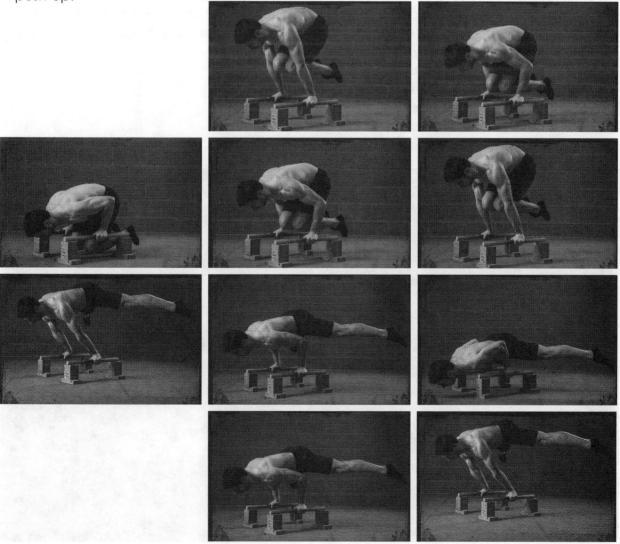

Front Lever

Although the pulling exercises we looked at in Chapter 6 are very useful and build unreal amounts of strength, they all have one commonality; the pull was initiated and performed with bent arms. Pulling with straight arms is completely different and in most cases much more difficult. This is where the front lever comes in. The front lever is almost entirely unknown outside the gymnastics and climbing community, but is one of the best tests of pulling and core strength out there. It is similar in concept to the back lever, except that the body position is reversed. This movement is much more difficult than the back lever as the shoulder joint is free to rotate, whilst in the back lever it is not. As with all of the other lever movements in this chapter, make sure that your elbows remain locked at all times. This dramatically reduces the leverage you will be able to exert on the movement, building more strength and a more impressive physique. You should also use an overhand grip for all stages.

As the front lever is a static hold, we cannot do the traditional sets and repetitions normally done with any other exercise, so we will use the same method as for the planche. This involves holding the position for a set amount of time in as many sets as it takes you. For example, if the target time is 30 seconds, and you can only hold the position for 5 seconds, you would perform 6 sets of 5 seconds to equal the 30-second total.

As before, your hold times will increase as you become stronger, so that you will do 3 sets of 10 seconds, 2 sets of 15 seconds, and then the entire 30 seconds in one go. Once you can hold the position for 30 seconds in a single set, move onto the next stage.

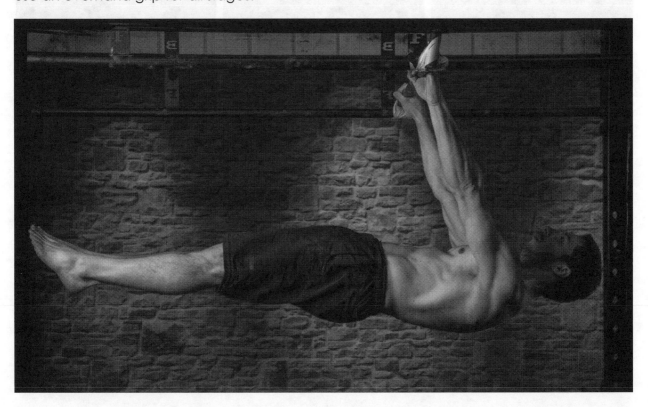

Vertical Pulls

The most difficult aspect of the front lever, barring the extreme stress on the core, is the fact that throughout the whole movement the arms must stay completely locked out. It is this action that allows such high pulling strength to be built and makes the front lever so beneficial. Pulling with straight arms is a very difficult concept for many people to adapt to, as the body will nearly always want to bend the elbows to make the movement easier and to protect the elbow joints from damage. To learn this, we can perform an exercise called vertical pulls. They will familiarise you with pulling down with straight arms, and they will also teach you to "lock in" the scapula, as was taught in the shoulder mobility section (Chapter 4).

1. Grab a pull-up bar with an overhand grip, shoulder width apart, and hang with completely straight arms.

2. From here, pull your scapulae down. To do this, think about moving your shoulders down and away from your ears.

3. Then start to pull down with your hands, as if you are trying to pull them down through the bar. You should be trying to reduce the angle at your armpit as much as possible. Lean back into it and allow the lower body to stay limp.

4. Hold this position for as long as you can, making sure that your form is correct. Try and hold the position for 30 seconds, in as many sets as it takes you. Once you can hold the position for 30 seconds continuously, move onto the next stage.

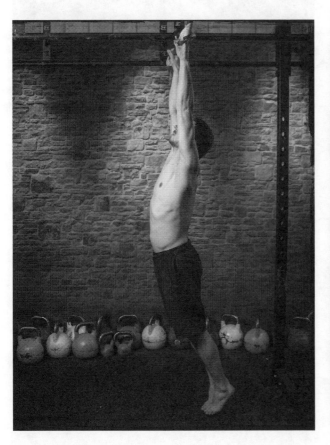
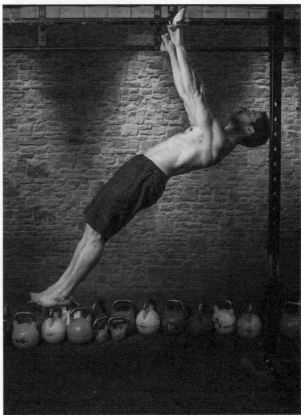

Tuck Front Lever

Once you have practiced the vertical pulls and you have an idea of what it feels like to pull down with straight arms, you can move onto this stage, which is the first actual front lever position you will perform. The tuck front lever has exactly the same upper body position as the proper version, but the core and the legs are tucked up tight to keep the bodyweight as close to the hands as possible. There is no other requirement here other than to have the hips and shoulders level with each other, so do not worry if your back is rounded.

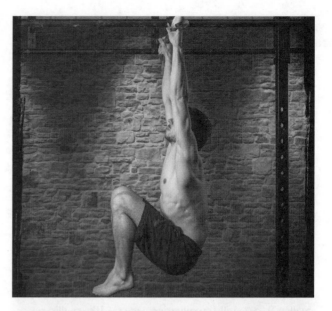

1. Grab the bar with an overhand grip. Your hands should be shoulder width apart.

2. Tuck your knees up to your chest (as in the hanging knee raise), and pull down as hard as you can. Keep pulling your hips up until they become level with your shoulders.

3. Now hold this position for as long as you can.

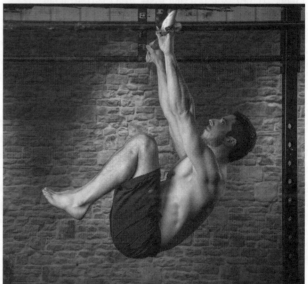

Teaching Points

At first, you may struggle to pull your body up at all. To help with this, kick off the ground and use momentum to get into the tuck position. As you become stronger, you will be able to use less momentum and more pulling strength.

Aim to hold this for a total of 30 seconds, in as many sets as it takes you. Once you can hold the position for 30 seconds continuously, move onto the next stage.

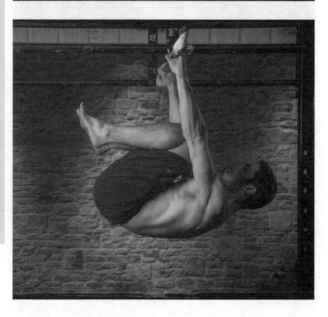

Flat Back Front Lever

Once you are confident with the tuck front lever, you can move onto the flat back variation. Whereas the tuck front lever allowed a rounded back, the flat back variation does not. Although the two exercises may look almost identical, the flattening of the lower back is extremely difficult for a couple of reasons:

- Firstly, flattening the back makes the front of the core and the abdominals longer, which means that they must fight harder to exert any force.

- Secondly, flattening the back moves more of your bodyweight away from your hands, which forces the back muscles to work even harder to maintain the position.

1. Get into a tuck front lever.

2. Now attempt to lower your hips and flatten your back. It should feel like you are trying to tilt your pelvis forwards, or stick your butt out. Do not let your elbows bend.

3. You will reach the correct position when your hips are level with your shoulders and your entire back is as flat as you can make it. Now hold this position for as long as you can.

Teaching Points

As has been said, this exercise only looks slightly different from the tuck front lever, but is actually much more challenging. It is quite likely that you will not be able to hold the position for any length of time at first, so to build strength, allow your back to become flat for a split second and then allow it to curve. As your strength increases, so will your hold times.

As this position is more difficult than the one before, you should aim to hold this for a total of 20 seconds, in as many sets as it takes you. Once you can hold the position for 20 seconds continuously, move onto the next stage.

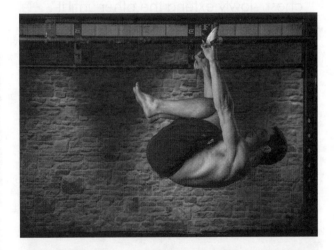

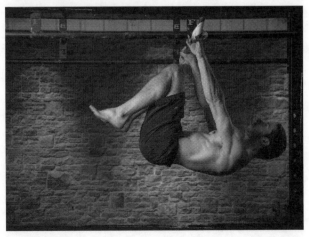

Single-Leg Front Lever

Once you can hold the tuck front lever with a flat back, the next stage is to start extending one of your legs to achieve the single-leg front lever. This movement has one leg completely straight whilst the other is tucked up into the chest. Although this sounds much more difficult than the previous stage, it actually isn't. This is because the leg that is tucked up into the chest keeps a lot of the bodyweight underneath the hands, whilst the straight leg can help to generate tension in the rest of the body, helping to hold the position for longer.

1. Grab the bar with an overhand grip and get into the flat back front lever position.

2. Keeping one leg tucked tightly into your chest, slowly extend the other until it becomes completely straight. Point the toes of your straight leg to help generate muscular tension, and do not let your elbows bend.

3. Hold this position for as long as you can. Make sure you perform sets with each leg extended so as not to create any strength imbalances.

Teaching Points

Having said that this movement is no more difficult than the previous stage. The act of extending your leg will place a much greater demand on your core than the previous variations, so take your time and do not get frustrated if you struggle to perform it correctly. Being diligent and maintaining good form is the best method here. If you extend a leg and your hips begin to bend then bring the leg back in a small amount.

Aim to hold this for a total of 20 seconds, in as many sets as it takes you. Once you can hold the position for 20 seconds continuously, move onto the next stage.

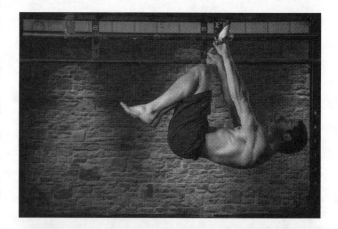

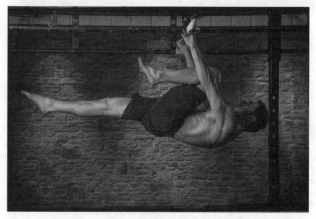

Straddle Front Lever

Once you have some experience with single-leg front levers, you can start working on extending both legs at the same time in a straddle "V" position. This variation is much more challenging than the single-leg version as your core has to fully support the entire weight of your lower body with your hips in a completely open position. If you have a flexible lower body, then this movement will be easier for you, as a wider straddle or "V" shape will mean that more of your bodyweight is closer to your hands, which makes the exercise easier. If you find that you are really struggling, it pays to spend some time working on your flexibility.

There a two ways to arrive in the straddle front lever and both of them can be beneficial. In my experience, it is best to use both methods as they can really help you to break through sticking points and plateaus. The methods are:

• From a tuck front lever
• Pendulums

As the straddle front lever is extremely difficult, aim to hold it for a total of 10 seconds, in as many sets as it takes you. Once you can hold the position for 10 seconds continuously, move onto the final stage.

1. From a Tuck Front Lever

The first method of getting into the straddle front lever is to move from one of the tuck variations and then slowly extend both legs. This requires a lot of control and muscular tension, and is perhaps the most difficult way to move into the position, but it looks the smoothest and strongest.

1. Get into the tuck front lever position.

2. From here, start to slowly extend your legs into a wide straddle "V" position. As the weight of your legs moves away from your centre of mass, you will have to pull down progressively harder.

3. Keep moving your legs out until your entire body is horizontal. Now hold this position for as long as you can.

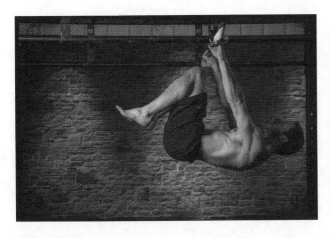

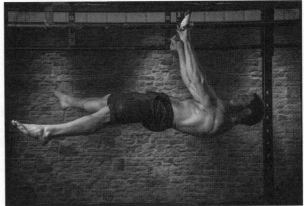

2. Pendulums

The second and perhaps most impressive way to get into a straddle front lever is by using pendulums. The pendulum is simply a way of getting the body into the correct position by using momentum, and allows you to keep the strict body position throughout the entire movement.

1. Grab a pull-up bar with an overhand grip and pull your chin over the bar.

2. From here, aim to swing your legs forwards but move your shoulders back and down until you reach the horizontal position. At first it may seem difficult to lock out your elbows at the bottom of the movement but keep practicing and it will come.

3. Hold the horizontal position for as long as you can. At first this may only be a split second, but with time and practice your strength will increase.

4. When you cannot hold the position any longer, pull yourself back up to the top of the pull-up by letting your lower body swing back underneath you and pulling your shoulders up and forwards. As you progress simply remain in the horizontal position for longer.

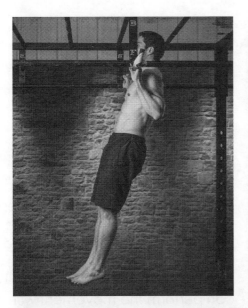
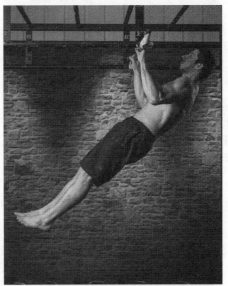
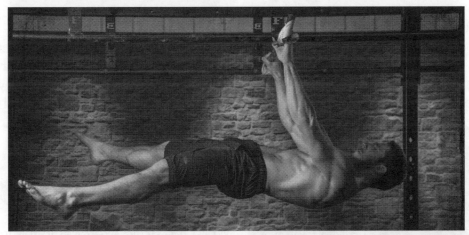
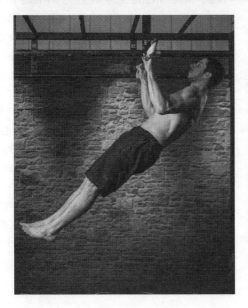
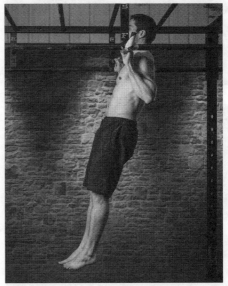

Full Front Lever

Once you have built up the necessary strength working with the straddle front lever, you can start to bring the legs together to achieve a true front lever. This is fractionally more difficult than the straddle variation, although some people report that having the legs together enables them to generate more tension in the body.

1. Grab the bar with an overhand grip, and get into a straddle front lever.

2. Now bring both of your legs together until they are touching and completely straight. Point your toes and try and generate as much tension as possible throughout your entire body. Do not allow your elbows to bend.

3. Hold this position and do not allow your hips to bend.

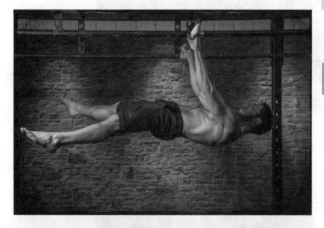

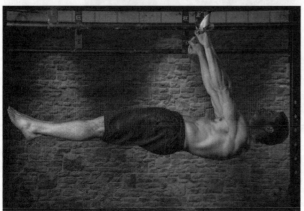

Teaching Points

In addition to the method just described, you can use either of the two methods demonstrated for getting into the front lever position: *from a tuck front lever* and *pendulums*. Keep working with it until you can perform the movement with good form.

As this variation is extremely difficult, aim to hold it for a total of 10 seconds, in as many sets as it takes you. Try and work your way up to a continuous hold time of 10 seconds.

Front Lever Pull-up

Whilst the static exercises in this front lever section are excellent for developing strength, if you are looking for an additional challenge or just a bit more variety, you can start training front lever pull-ups. To do this, simply assume the front lever position of your choice, and perform a pull-up. For these to be maximally effective, ensure that you maintain a good form throughout. This includes locking out the elbow at the bottom of every repetition. As an example, shown below is a tuck front lever pull-up. As the front lever pull-up is much more difficult than normal pull-ups, aim to do 3 sets of 3 to 5 repetitions.

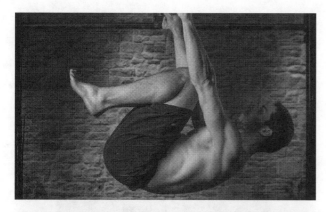

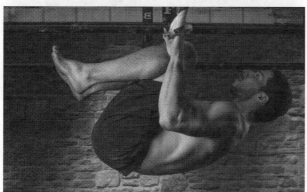

Back Lever

The third lever-type exercise that we are going to look at in this chapter is the back lever. This can be thought of as the complete opposite of the front lever, as it works many of the opposing muscle groups. It is also extremely useful for developing strength for the planche: in fact, in my experience, I would say that a solid back lever is a prerequisite for a good planche. Traditionally, a gymnast uses the back lever when manoeuvering in and out of strength positions on the rings. It also prepares the athlete to exert strength in an unnatural or mechanically disadvantaged position.

The back lever can be performed with either an overhand grip or underhand grip. Using an overhand grip is easier, as there is much less stress on the biceps and its associated tendons. However, if you perform the back lever with an underhand

grip, you will develop awesome biceps and elbow strength, which is vital for planche training with fingers positioned backwards, and for more advanced gymnastic training, such as the Iron Cross. I would recommend using both grips, as this will ensure that you have all-round strength and are not weaker in one position than the other.

You will find that even though they are somewhat equal and opposite in terms of the muscles they use, the front lever and back lever are not equal in difficulty. In my experience the vast majority of people achieve their first proper back lever well before their first proper front lever. There are many reasons for this, the main ones being that the shoulder is in a naturally more inflexible position in the back lever, and that the muscles used in the back lever are traditionally stronger than those used in the front lever.

As with other exercises that have this level of difficulty, I have broken down the method of learning the back lever into several stages. Make sure that you are comfortable and confident enough with each stage before moving onto the next one.

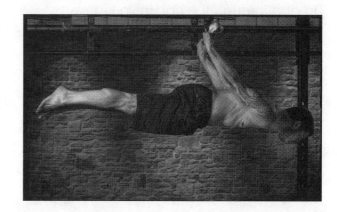

German Hang

The first stage in learning the back lever is the German hang. It will develop strength and flexibility in the shoulders and back, and prepare the body for the progressions towards the more difficult variations.

1. Grasp the pull-up bar with an overhand or underhand grip.

2. Keeping your elbows locked out, tuck your legs up to your chest and pull down hard. Aim to get your legs through the gap in the middle of your arms.

3. Keep rotating round until you are facing forwards again, and then extend your legs down to the floor. You are now in the German hang position. Simply hold this position for as long as you can, in order to build flexibility in the shoulder and for strength. Then let go and drop to the ground, or rotate back around by reversing the movement.

Teaching Points

When first trying to get into the German hang, you may struggle to pull your legs up and through the gap in your arms. Kicking up into this position from the floor can help, as can building your pulling strength with either pull-ups or the front lever. Strengthening your core will also help. Practice rotating forwards and backwards to become comfortable in this position; this will also build strength around the shoulder joint. Once you have become comfortable getting into and out of the German hang, it is time to start working on the next stage.

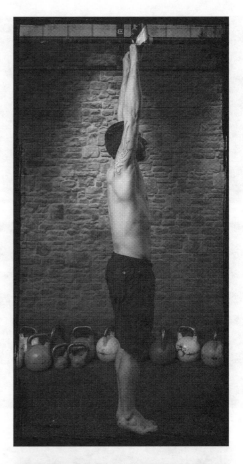

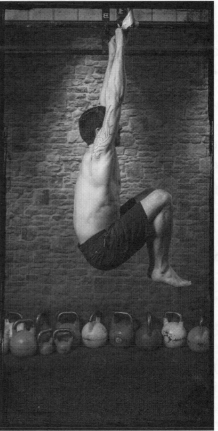

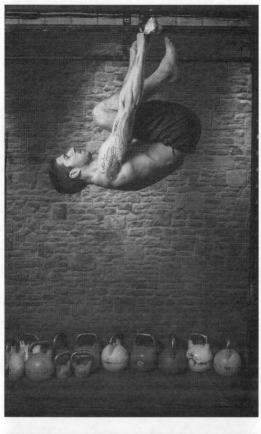
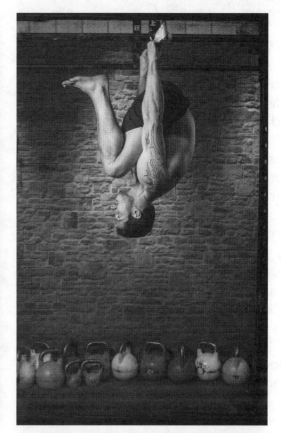
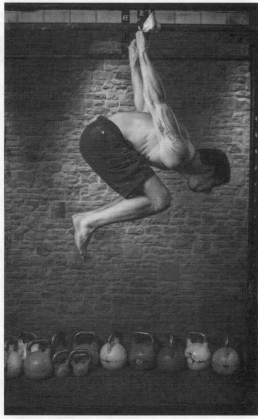
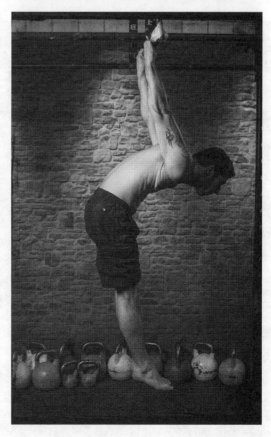

Tuck Back Lever

Once you have mastered the German hang, it is time to start raising the hips up to achieve the tuck back lever. This is not as difficult as the tuck front lever, and you should find that your progress is quite fast.

1. Grasp the pull-up bar with an overhand or underhand grip, and get into a German hang.

2. From this position, tuck your knees tightly into your chest and then raise your hips up until they are level with your shoulders. It is fine at this stage to have a rounded back. Make sure to lock out your elbows and pull down as hard as you can.

3. Once you are sure that your position is good, hold it for as long as you can.

Teaching Points

To generate strength in this unusual position, attempt to squeeze your arms together behind your back. This will help to generate the muscular tension needed to hold the position.

As with the other static positions, hold this for a total time of 20 seconds, in as many sets as it takes you. Once you can hold this variation for 20 seconds continuously, move onto the next stage.

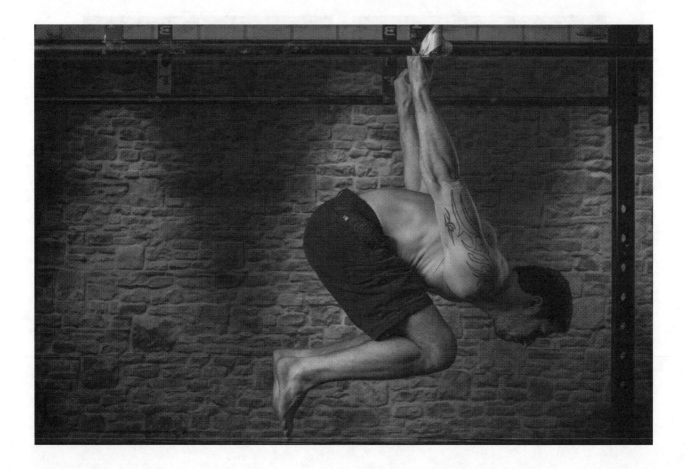

Flat Back Lever

As with the front lever, the next stage in the back lever is to flatten out the back and move the hips and lower body a little further away from the hands. This stage requires more muscular control and is much more challenging than the tuck variation. Simply put, in this stage you should be attempting to make your entire back as flat as possible.

1. Grasp the pull-up bar with an overhand or underhand grip, and get into a tuck back lever. Lock your arms into your sides and pull down as hard as you can.

2. From this position try to flatten out your back. This means that you have to make the abdominals longer whilst contracting the lower and middle back. Think about tilting your pelvis forwards (sticking your butt out) when you do this.

3. As soon as you reach the correct position, hold it for as long as you can.

Teaching Points

Flattening out the back can be very difficult, especially if you are new to these types of static exercises. To make this easier, you should move into the position for a split second and then move back into the tuck back lever position. Keep doing this whilst striving to hold the flat back position for increasing lengths of time.

Again, hold this position for 20 seconds, in as many sets as it takes you. Once you can hold the position for 20 seconds continuously, move onto the next stage.

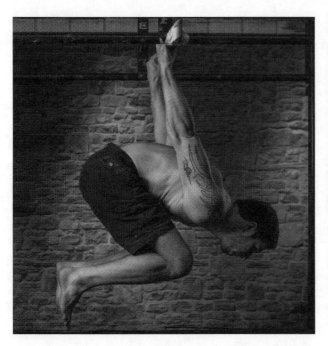
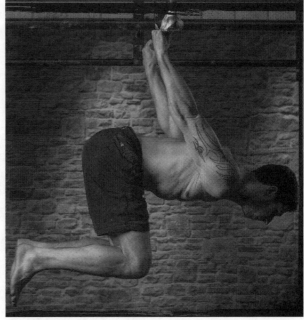

Single-Leg Back Lever

Once you are comfortable with the advanced tuck back lever, it is time to start extending your legs to move more of your bodyweight away from your hands. The single-leg back lever is not actually that much more difficult than the flat back lever, mainly because one leg will be tucked up tight into the chest, which keeps a lot of your bodyweight close to your hands.

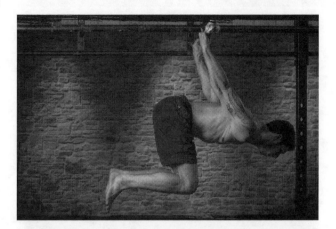

1. Grasp the bar or rings with an overhand or underhand grip, and get into a flat back lever.

2. Tuck one leg tightly into your chest, then start to move one leg out behind you until it is straight. Point your toes to help align your body and generate muscular tension.

3. Now hold this position for as long as you can.

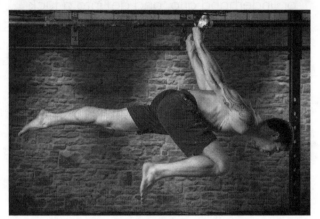

Teaching Points

If you cannot extend your leg out behind you until it is straight, just move it as far as you are able. As you become stronger, you will be able to extend it further each time. Make sure to work both legs equally to ensure that no strength imbalances occur.

Again, hold this position for 20 seconds, in as many sets as it takes you. Once you can hold the position for 20 seconds continuously, move onto the next stage.

Straddle Back Lever

Once you have mastered the single-leg back lever, both legs can start to be extended at the same time to arrive at a straddle back lever. This is a vital stage, as once you have mastered this you will be able to start bringing the legs together to achieve a full back lever.

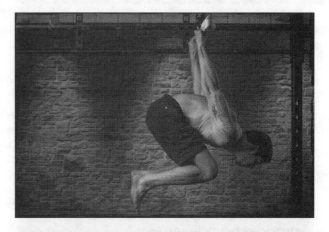

1. Grasp the bar or rings with an overhand or underhand grip, and get into a flat back lever.

2. From this position, extend both legs in a wide straddle "V" position. The wider the straddle the easier the movement will be. Point your toes to generate muscular tension and align your body.

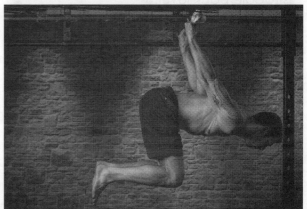

3. Now hold this position for as long as you can.

Teaching Points

You should be aiming to hold the position for 20 seconds in as many sets as it takes you. Once you can hold the position for 20 seconds continuously, move onto the next stage.

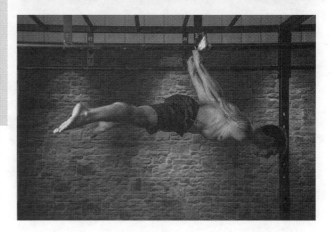

Full Back Lever

Once you can hold the straddle back lever for 20 seconds in a single set, it will be time for you to move onto the full back lever. This is where the legs are brought together until the body forms a completely straight line. This is a more challenging position to hold, but is essential to achieve if you want to progress with the planche.

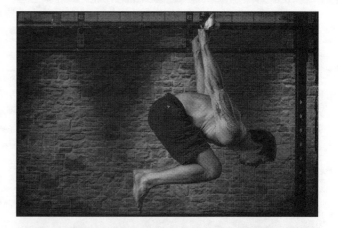

1. Grasp the bar or rings with an overhand or underhand grip, and get into a straddle back lever.

2. From this position, bring your legs together until they are touching. Point your toes and contract all the muscles in your lower body as hard as you can.

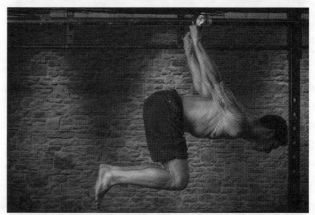

3. Hold this position for as long as you are able.

Teaching Points

If you find that you cannot hold the position for long, bring your legs together for a second, then widen them to a straddle again. Keep doing this until your hold times increase.

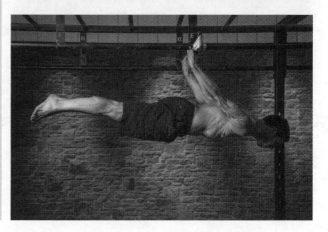

As this is a very strenuous position, don't worry if you cannot hold it for a total of 20 seconds. A continuous hold time of 10 to 15 seconds is still impressive.

Half Lever

The half lever is the simplest of the gymnastic core exercises, and at first glance looks to be fairly straightforward. Once you attempt it however, you will appreciate just how demanding it is, and how easy most other core training is. The half lever is also called the "L sit" in gymnastic circles, and is one of the foundation exercises that all gymnasts must perfect if they are looking to build enough core strength to do well.

The half lever is also an absolutely perfect example of the disadvantaged leverage principle that was mentioned in the introduction. As the weight of the legs is moved further away from the hands, the core has to work progressively harder to support the lower body, which is why this exercise builds so much strength without having to add any external weight.

The half lever is also one of the handful of movements we have looked at so far (along with the planche, front lever, and back lever), that relies on performing hold times instead of the traditional sets and repetitions. As with the other exercises, you should be looking to hold the position for a specific total time in as many sets as it takes you. For the half lever, I recommend building up to a total hold time of at least 30 seconds.

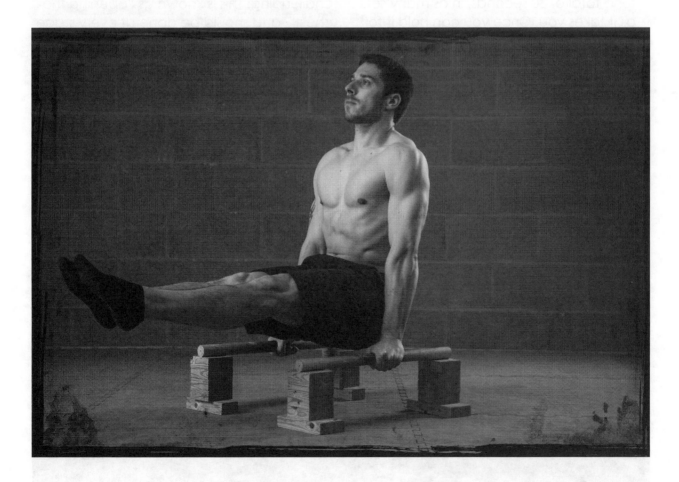

Tuck Half Lever

The aim of this first stage in learning the half lever is to hold a simplified position where the legs do not have to be fully extended. You can use anything to help you with this, including chairs, boxes, aerobic steps, or any other raised platform. I personally use parallettes.

1. Place your hands on your chosen platform and lock out your elbows.

2. Push down hard and then raise your legs until your thighs are horizontal. You should keep a 90-degree bend in the knee.

3. Now simply hold this position for as long as you can. You should aim to hold this for a total of 30 seconds, in as many sets as it takes you. Once you can hold it for 30 seconds continuously, move onto the next stage.

Teaching Points

Although the tuck half lever is difficult enough by itself, as soon as you are able to, you should start trying to push your hips as far forwards as you can. This action makes the angle between your legs and torso wider, making the movement more challenging. This is known as "opening the chest", and should be done at every stage of your half lever training in order to build as much core strength as possible.

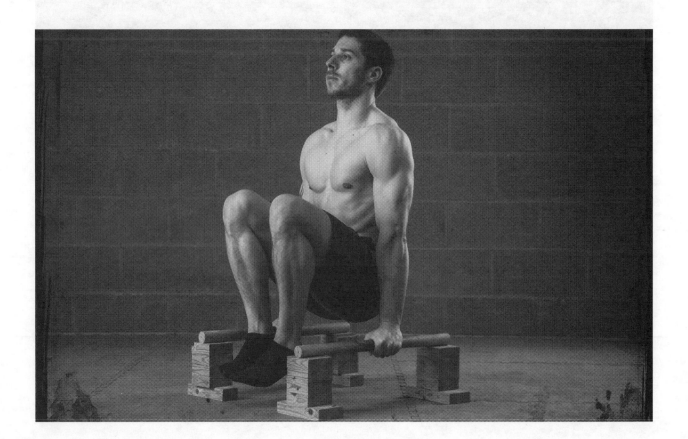

Angled Half Lever

Once you have built up some core strength with the tuck variation, you can start to work with the angled half lever. This involves straightening out the legs whilst keeping them below the level of your hands. Again, you will need to use some sort of platform for your hands to rest on.

1. Place your hands on your chosen platform and lock out your elbows.

2. Push down hard with your arms and then straighten your legs out in front of you so that your heels are an inch or two above the floor. Try and get the legs into a 45-degree angle. Remember to keep your knees locked out if you can, or bend your knees if you can't.

3. Now hold this position for as long as you can. You should aim to hold this for a total of 30 seconds, in as many sets as it takes you. Once you can hold it for 30 seconds continuously, move onto the next stage.

Teaching Points

If this stage is too difficult for you, try using a higher platform for your hands. This will allow your legs to still be straight, but your core will not have to work as hard as more of your lower body's weight will be closer to your hands. Make the movement as easy as you need to in order for you to be able to perform it properly. Form is everything here, and better form will mean quicker progress and better results. Again, as with the tuck variation, start pushing your hips forwards as soon as possible.

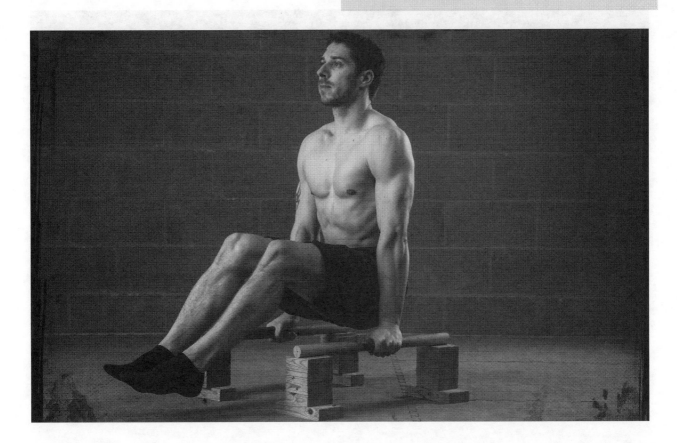

Half Lever

Once you have mastered the raised half lever, you can start working on raising your legs up until they are horizontal. This stage can take some time, but is made easier if you follow the progressions that I have laid out. It is also worth saying that breathing in the half lever is always somewhat difficult, as the diaphragm, which is a core muscle used for inflating and deflating the lungs, can start to act as a stabiliser if the movement is very difficult. Try and take small breaths when performing all of the half lever variations.

1. Place your hands on the platform that you are using and lock out your elbows.

2. Push down hard with your arms and raise your legs up until they are horizontal. Keep your knees locked and point your toes to generate muscular tension.

3. Try and hold this position for as long as you can. Again, as with the other variations, you should aim to hold this for a total of 30 seconds, in as many sets as it takes you. Once you can hold it for 30 seconds continuously, move onto the final stage.

Teaching Points

As the half lever is so difficult, you will probably not be able to hold the position for very long before your legs drop. To spend time in the position and to build strength, move your legs out into the full position quickly, before bringing them back in until you arrive in the tuck half lever position. Continue doing this and your hold times will steadily increase.

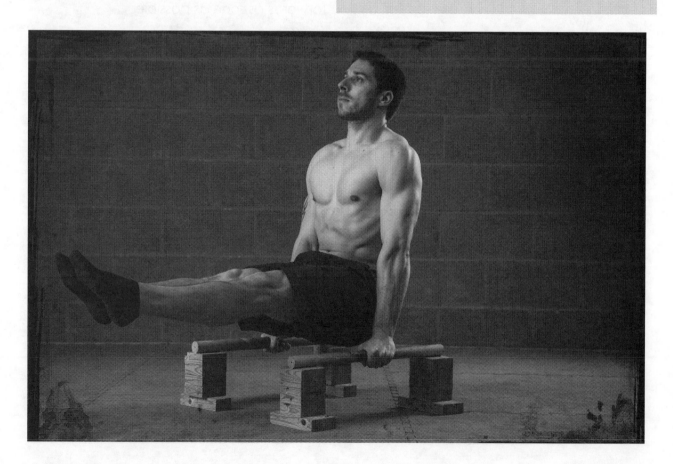

Floor Half Lever

Once you have achieved the half lever using a platform of some kind, it will be time for you to try and start performing it using nothing more than the floor. This is much more difficult as you need to ensure that you are pushing down as hard as possible, and also that your legs are high enough and horizontal enough for them not to drop to the ground.

1. Sit down with completely straight legs. Place your hands on the ground next to your hips and lock out your elbows.

2. From here, push down with your arms as hard as you can. Attempt to draw your scapulae down to help elevate your entire body. At the same time, lift your legs from the floor and extend them straight out in front of you. Point your toes to generate muscular tension.

3. Now hold this position for as long as you can. Again, as with the other variations, you should aim to hold this for a total of 30 seconds, in as many sets as it takes you.

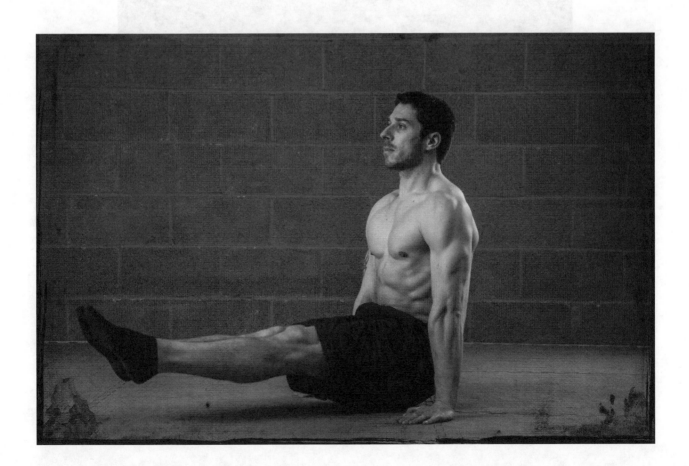

Half Lever Extensions

After you have spent some time with the half lever, you can start to add some movement into the exercise to make it a little more exciting and challenging. Half lever extensions are the simplest way, and can help us to learn how to push the hips forwards and open up the chest. You should be aiming to increase the angle at the hips as much as possible with these.

1. Get into a tucked half lever with your knees held tightly into the chest.

2. From here, extend both of your legs out at the same time until they are completely straight.

3. As soon as they are straight, keep extending and try and push the hips as far forwards as you can, then retract both of your legs until your knees are tucked tightly into your chest again. This counts as one repetition. Try and perform as many repetitions as possible in 30 seconds.

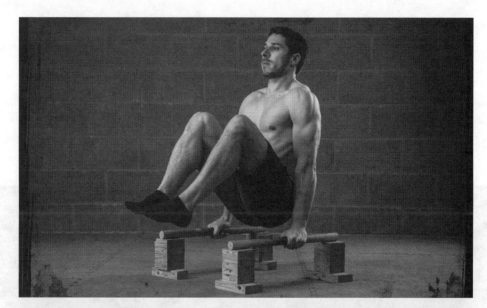

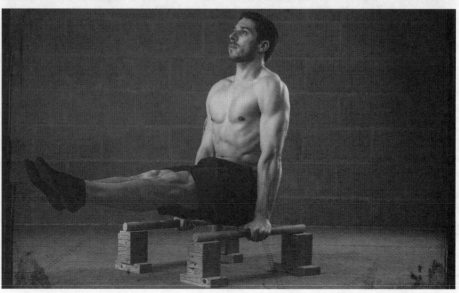

Half Lever Bicycles

Another excellent variation that we can use to make the half lever more interesting and more challenging is to move each leg out to full extension one at a time. I have called these 'half lever bicycles'.

1. Get into a half lever, but have one leg tucked into the chest and the other fully extended.

2. Now bring the extended leg back in towards your chest whilst extending the other. Hold each position for a second or two before continuing. Try and perform as many repetitions as possible in 30 seconds.

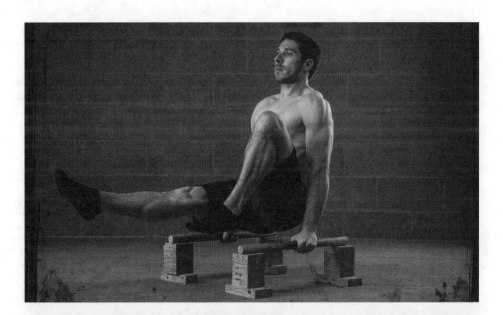

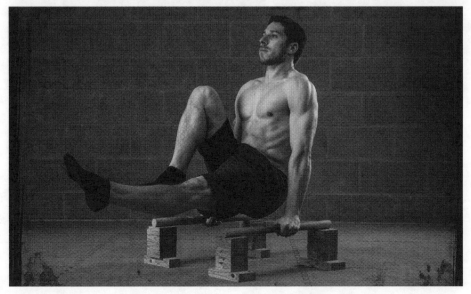

Half Lever Swimmers

The last variation of the half lever that you can add to your training is the half lever swimmer. This is simply the half lever position held either on the floor or on a raised platform, with a swimming action by the legs. This really helps to work the core as much as possible.

1. Get into a normal half lever position either on the floor or supported on parallettes or a raised platform.

2. From here, simply lower one leg towards the ground whilst raising the other into the air. Then lower the raised leg and raise the lowered leg as many times as you can in a swimming action. Try and perform as many repetitions as possible in 30 seconds.

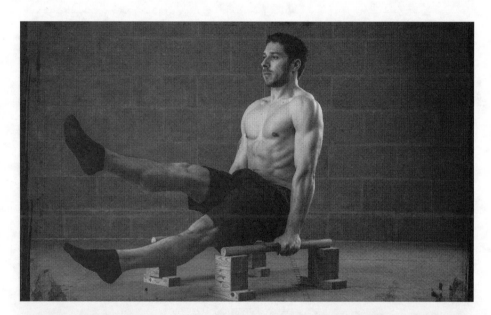

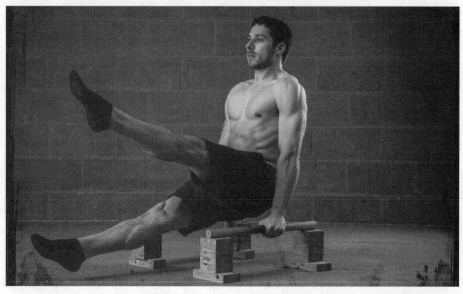

Human Flag

The human flag is another exercise that is excellent for all-over body strength, and places a huge demand on the oblique muscles of the torso. It combines pushing, pulling, and core strength and, above all else, looks extremely cool! It is also a very good exercise for developing straight-arm pulling and pushing strength in the upper body, as in the full version, one arm will be pushing as hard as possible whilst the other will be pulling as hard as possible. Many high-level athletes, e.g. Chinese Olympic weightlifters, also use this exercise.

To perform the human flag you will need a vertical pole or other suitable location. You will have to experiment to find a place that you can use regularly. I sometimes use a smith machine, squat rack, or even a climbing frame in the park. It is also advisable to use chalk to improve your grip, because if you struggle to hold on to the bar, you will have a real problem developing enough tension to complete the movement.

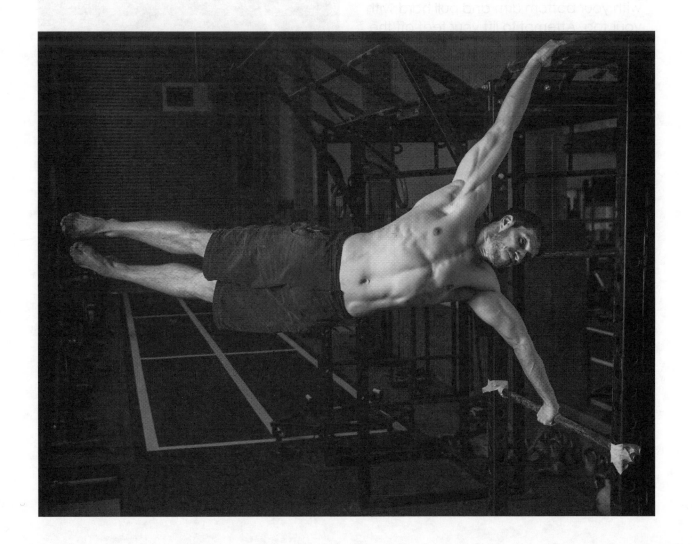

Vertical Flag

To start training the human flag you need to be able to hold your body vertically with straight arms. This stage is surprisingly difficult, and will hopefully give you an idea of what it is like to start training the flag.

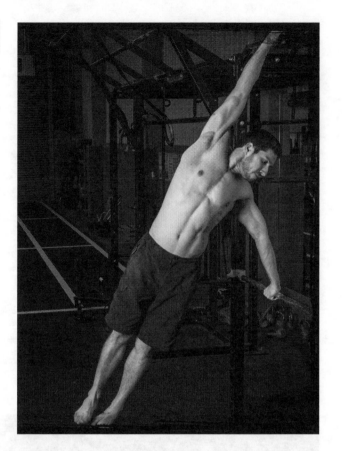

1. Grasp the bar(s) in the following way: the bottom hand with your fingers pointing down, palm facing away from you, and the top hand with your palm facing away. Your hands should be wider than shoulder width apart. You will just have to experiment here until you find a suitable and comfortable hand position.

2. Making sure that your elbows stay locked during the entire movement, push hard with your bottom arm and pull hard with your top. Attempt to lift your feet off the floor and hold your body vertically for as long as possible.

3. Make sure that you work both sides equally. This will ensure that you do not develop any strength imbalances.

Teaching Points

In terms of the hold times for this particular movement, as the flag is so difficult, you should aim for a total time of 10 to 15 seconds or so, in as many sets as it takes you. Once you can perform the exercise for the total time in one set, then move onto the next stage.

Tucked Flag

Once you have got used to the vertical flag, it is time to start trying to raise the torso into a more horizontal position. Obviously, the further out we stick our legs the more difficult the movement, so for the second stage we are going to keep our legs and knees tucked up into the chest as much as possible.

1. Grasp the bar the way it was described above. Jump your feet off the floor and tuck your knees up to your chest. At the same time push hard with your bottom arm and pull hard with the top.

2. Keep pushing and pulling hard with both arms until your torso is horizontal.

3. Try and hold this position for as long as possible. Make sure you work both sides equally.

Teaching Points

Again, you should aim for a total time of 10 to 15 seconds or so, in as many sets as it takes you. Once you can perform the exercise for the total time in one set, then move onto the next stage.

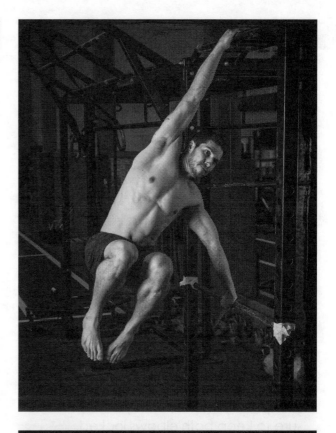

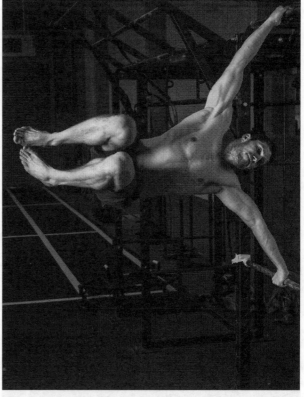

Straddle Flag

Once you have built up a decent level of strength using the first and second stages, we can begin to extend the legs out from the body. This will make the movement much more challenging, as the leverage we can exert on the exercise is gradually reduced. The straddle flag requires you to position your legs in a wide "V" position, as this still allows some of your bodyweight to be close to the bar, but gives you an idea of what it is like to be in a correct flag position.

1. Grasp the bar in the usual way. Jump your feet up into the air and move them into the widest straddle you can.

2. Push down hard with your bottom arm, and pull down hard with your top. Make sure to keep both elbows locked.

3. Hold this position for as long as possible. Make sure you work both sides equally.

Teaching Points

The straddle flag is much more difficult than the tuck flag, and for this reason many people find it very challenging. To compensate for this I like to jump into the position with as much force as possible. This allows you to instantly arrive in the straddle flag position and try and sense what kind of strength it requires. In my journey with the flag this was the method that helped me the most, as it allowed my strength to develop slowly and also allowed me to work with the negative phase of the movement.

Again, you should aim for a total time of 10 to 15 seconds, in as many sets as it takes you. Once you can perform the exercise for the total time in one set, then move onto the final stage.

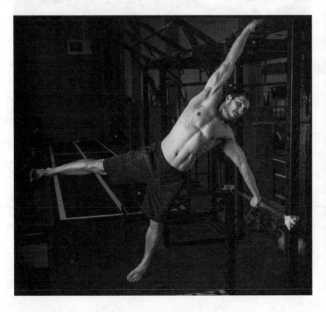

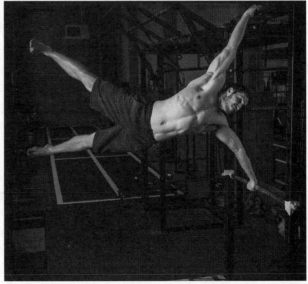

Human Flag

Once the straddle flag becomes easier, we can attempt to move into the proper human flag position where the legs are held together and the body is complete horizontal. Again, going from the straddle position to legs together is very intense, so take your time.

1. Start in the vertical or straddle flag position.

2. From the vertical flag, push and pull hard until you reach a horizontal position. From the straddle flag, slowly bring your legs together. You can also jump into the position the same as before. Pointing your toes will help to contract your muscles and maintain the position.

3. Hold this for as long as possible. Again, make sure you work both sides equally.

Teaching Points

Again, you should aim for a total time of 10 to 15 seconds, in as many sets as it takes you. Perform the exercise for the total time in one set.

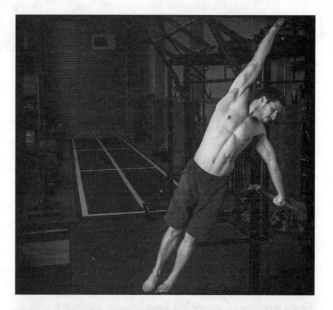

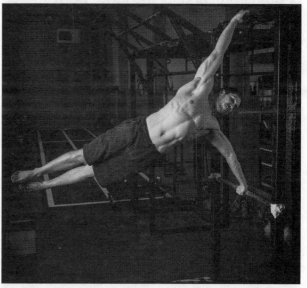

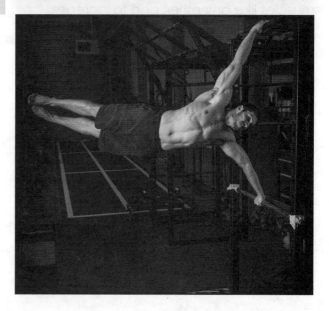

Although it may look like the upper body is king when it comes to calisthenics, the real workhorse muscle group is actually the core. The trunk or torso houses all of the muscles that act to stabilise the spine, and it is also the link between the upper body and lower body. A simple glance at exercises like the planche or the front lever should reinforce why the core is so important in these types of high-level movements. The core acts as a home point or foundation for the upper body to pull or push from, and for the lower body to jump, squat and leap from. As an athlete you could have the strongest upper body and lower body on the planet, but if you cannot connect them with a strong core, then it won't perform to its maximum potential.

Traditionally the core has been trained with crunches, sit-ups, and other movements that are more suited for many repetitions. Who hasn't heard of some celebrity or other boasting about how they do 1000 crunches a day? Whilst this may be good for their egos, it is next to useless for developing strength. The core muscles are muscles like any other, and to increase strength, the resistance that they contract against has to increase with time. However, the core is not a body part like the arms or legs. The arms and legs can perform a wide variety of tasks, e.g. move around in different directions, as well as grab or hold onto bars and other objects, etc. The core is unable to do these dynamic activities, so building strength in the core may appear more challenging.

As usual, the key to developing strength using bodyweight exercises and calisthenics lies in knowing *what* exercises to perform and *how* to perform them. You will remember the principle of decreased leverage that I talked about in the introduction; well, this is where that principle really comes into play. As we cannot add weight to the core, and as we are not using any machines or other elaborate equipment, we will use decreased leverage to progressively make the exercises in the core section increasingly challenging, so that eventually you can build an absolutely bombproof core. Do not be under any illusions; once you can perform some of the more advanced exercises in this chapter, you will have more core strength than you ever thought possible.

As a last note, doing core work alone will not develop a six-pack, no matter what you have been told by various fitness "experts". Burning fat off one area of the body in particular, known as "spot reducing", does not and cannot happen: the only factors that truly work if you wish to reduce your body fat are a good diet and a good conditioning regime.

Plank

The first core exercise that we are going to look at in this chapter, and the one that most people are familiar with, is the plank. As the name suggests, this exercise requires you to hold your body in a rigid, "plank-like" position, for as long as you can. This is another static or isometric exercise so we will not be performing sets and repetitions here, but hold times instead.

1. Place either your forearms or your hands on the floor as you would for a push-up. Stretch your feet out behind you and balance on your toes.

2. Now raise your hips up until your shoulders, hips, knees, and ankles are in line. Hold this position for as long as possible.

Teaching Points

One of the biggest issues for many people starting with the plank is that they have an arch in the lower back. This will be seen as a hollow shape where the back meets the hips, and is a sign of weakness in the core. It is also common for women to have an exaggerated hollow, simply because of their body shape and bone structure. To rectify this, try and squeeze your abdominals as hard as possible and tuck your butt underneath your hips. This should act to flatten out the lower back and is a stronger position. In terms of hold times, initially try and hold the position for 3 sets of 20 seconds. As this becomes easier, increase the hold times for as long as you can.

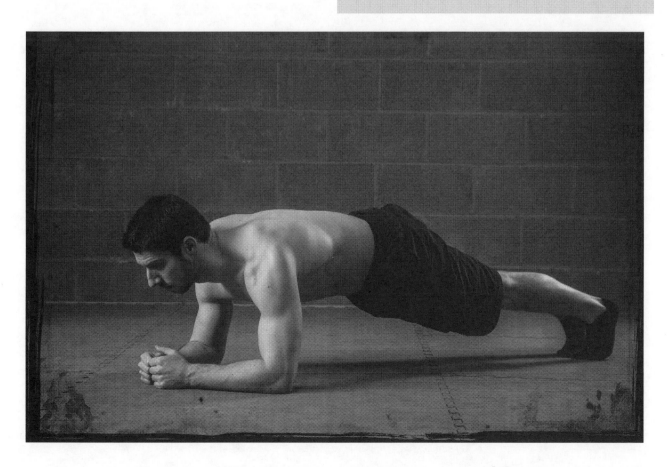

Side Plank

The side plank is the gateway to the oblique group of exercises, and is almost exactly the same as the plank, just in a different body orientation. Again, this is a static exercise, so that means that you will perform the movement for a set hold time instead of sets and repetitions.

1. Place one forearm on the ground and stretch out your legs at 90 degrees to this arm.

2. Place your bottom foot on its side, and position your other foot on top.

3. Now raise your hips up until a straight line can be drawn through your shoulders, hips, knees, and ankles. Your torso should be square on to the ground and you should feel tension in your obliques closest to the ground.

4. Now hold this position for as long as possible. Be sure to switch sides and work the opposite oblique as well.

Teaching Points

In terms of hold times, initially try and hold the position for 3 sets of 20 seconds. As this becomes easier, increase the hold times for as long as you can.

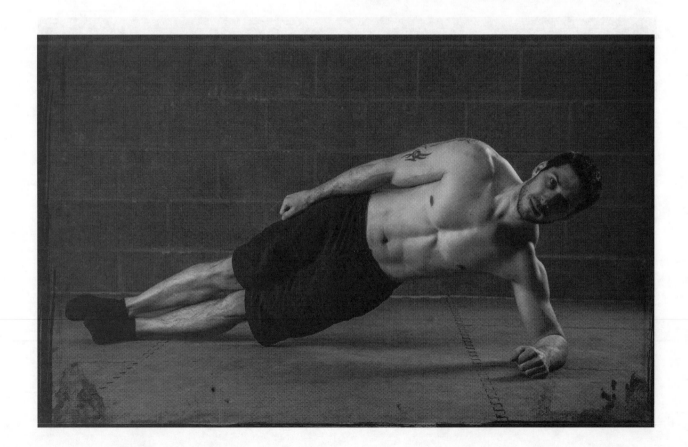

Crunch

Although I mentioned the crunch in derogatory terms in the introduction to this chapter, it is nevertheless a useful exercise with which to build a little core strength. This is easily achievable by the majority of people, even if they have no training history whatsoever.

1. Lie on your back with your knees bent at around 90 degrees and your feet flat on the floor. You may wish to tuck your toes under something solid to stop them moving.

2. Cross your arms and fold them in front of your chest.

3. From here, curl your shoulders and upper back off the ground and move your chest towards your knees. Stop when your upper and middle back are off the ground, and do not allow your lower back to come off the floor.

4. Finally lower your shoulders down to the ground. This counts as one repetition.

Teaching Points

You should be able to crank out a fair number of sets and repetitions because of the simple nature of this exercise: aim for 3 to 4 sets of at least 20 repetitions. Once you can do this many, simply increase the number as far as you feel comfortable.

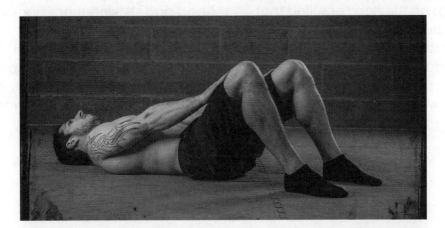

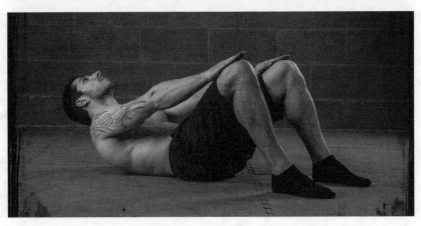

Dish

After looking at the two previous exercises, which are quite simple in nature and well known in the exercise community, this next one is a little less well known and can be much more difficult. The dish is very common in gymnastic circles, and is both an exercise and a body position. The name originates from the shape in which the body is held, being a shallow "U" shape, similar to an actual dish. It engages and requires the use of all of the abdominal muscles, and also teaches you to keep the spine in a stable position, which is a necessary skill for many of the other high-level calisthenic movements.

1. Lie on your back with your legs straight and your arms by your sides. Lift your shoulders and upper back off the floor, and lift your hands off the ground.

2. Lift your legs off the floor, ensuring that your lower back and middle back do not leave the ground. Think about pressing your spine down as hard as you can, or drawing your belly button towards the ground. Now hold this position for as long as possible.

Teaching Points

It will be almost impossible, for many people attempting the dish for the first time, to keep their entire back in contact with the ground for the duration of the exercise. To simplify the exercise, bend your knees and keep more of the weight of the legs closer to the torso. Then, as you become stronger, you can begin straightening the legs until they are completely locked out.

When you become comfortable performing the dish with your arms by your sides, you can increase the difficulty of the exercise and stretch the core out even further, by raising your arms above your head and sticking them back out behind you.

Initially try and hold this position for 3 sets of 10 seconds, and then steadily increase the hold times as you become stronger.

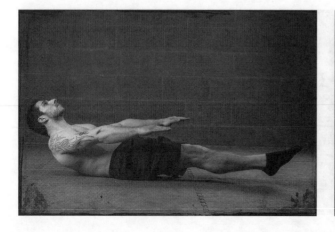
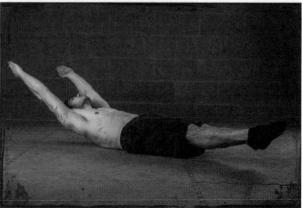

V-up

Once you have gained some experience performing the dish, we can add some movement to make it a little more interesting. The v-up is a combination of a dish, sit-up, and leg extension, and will test your strength, balance, and co-ordination.

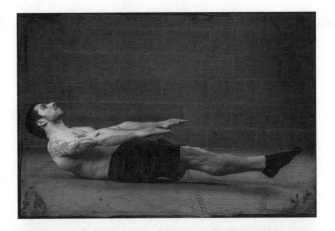

1. Get into the dish position with your arms by your sides.

2. From here, raise your torso off the ground, using your abdominals to do so.

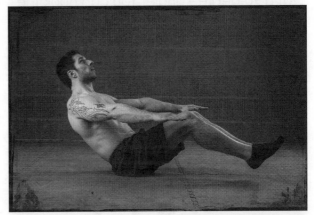

3. At the same time, bend your knees and bring your legs to your chest. Keep your arms stretched out in front to aid your balance, and try and keep your spine as straight as possible.

4. From this top position, reverse the movement until you reach the dish position once more. This counts as one repetition.

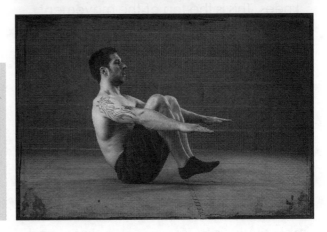

Teaching Points

Initially try and perform 3 sets of 10 repetitions, aiming to get as much control into the movement as possible. As this becomes easier, increase the number of repetitions to as many as you can.

Sit-up

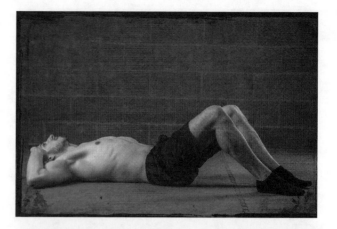

The sit-up is another well-known exercise, even to those who have not previously exercised or trained using calisthenics. It can be thought of as an extension of the crunch, and uses the core muscles, and to some extent the hip flexors, to lift the torso off the ground.

1. Lie on your back and position your knees at a 90-degree angle. You can hook the feet under something solid to help keep them on the ground. A training partner can also hold your ankles. Position your fingertips on your temples and lay your arms back so that your elbows touch the ground. This is the start position.

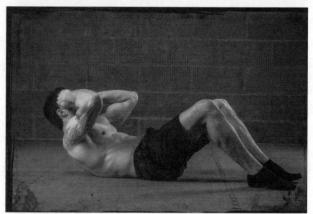

2. From here, contract your core muscles strongly and draw yourself up as far as you can. As you do so bring your elbows forwards until they touch or go over your knees. This is the top of the movement. From this position, lower yourself back down again to the start position. This counts as one repetition.

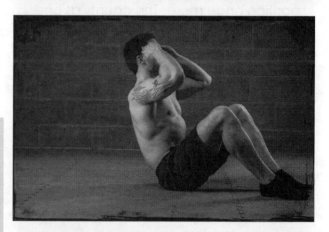

Teaching Points

For many people, sitting up fully and getting the elbows all of the way over the knees will be too difficult. To start with, simply sit up as far as you are able to, and as you become stronger, increase the range of motion until you can perform the movement properly.

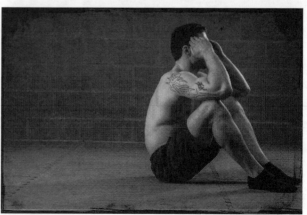

Initially try and do 3 sets of 20 repetitions, and then as you become stronger, increase the number of repetitions to as many as you can.

Lying Leg Extension

The lying leg extension is a mixture between the dish and the hanging knee raise, and the most efficient of the core exercises for targeting the lower abdominals. The main point to this movement, as with the dish, is to keep the lower and middle back pressed into the ground as hard as you can.

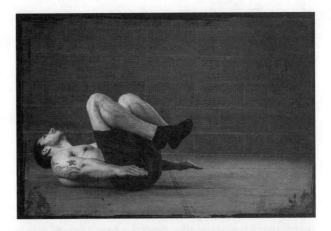

1. Lie on your back and lift your shoulders and upper back off the floor, as you did in the dish. Tuck your knees into your chest. This is the start position.

2. From here, start to extend your legs out until they become straight and the knees lock out. Keep your feet as close to the ground as you can all the way through the movement. Ensure that your entire spine stays firmly pressed into the ground at all times. From the extended position, bring your legs in slowly until they are tucked into your chest again. This counts as one repetition.

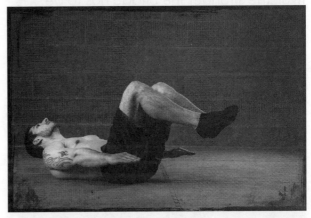

Teaching Points

As with the dish, if you find that your back comes away from the floor when you extend the legs, simply extend the legs out as far as you can until your back starts to come away from the ground. This will be the limit of your strength for that particular session. As you become stronger, you can extend the legs out further and further on each repetition.

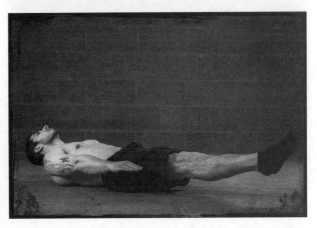

Start by doing 3 to 4 sets of 10 to 15 repetitions, and then increase the number of repetitions as you become stronger.

Extended Plank

The plank, which was the first exercise shown in this chapter, is good for beginners, and we can use a variation of it to build even more strength. To make the exercise more challenging, simply move the hands and feet further apart. This stretches out the core and forces it to become stronger to hold the position. A similar principle can be seen with bridges: the wider the span of a river, the stronger the bridge has to be.

1. Get into the push-up position.

2. Now start to walk the hands away from the feet, until you are in a stretched out position. Keep the lower back flat and the head looking down at the ground. Ideally you should keep moving the hands and feet further and further apart until your entire body is only a few inches from the floor.

3. Hold this position for as long as possible. Aim to make it challenging enough so that you fail at around 10 to 15 seconds.

Teaching Points

If you struggle to perform the extended plank with your whole body only a few inches from the ground, just walk your hands and feet as far apart as you can. As your strength increases, move them progressively further apart until you reach the end goal.

With the sets and repetitions here, the aim is to build as much strength as possible. This means that hold times of 30 seconds or so are not really worth it. You need to make the movement difficult enough so that you start to fail at around 10 seconds or so. If you find that you can carry on for more than 10 seconds, then move your hands and feet further apart. Doing 3 to 4 sets is also recommended.

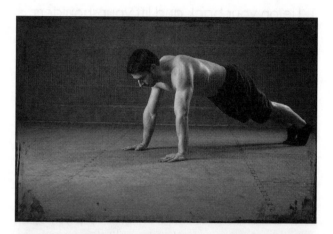

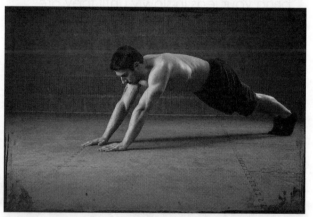

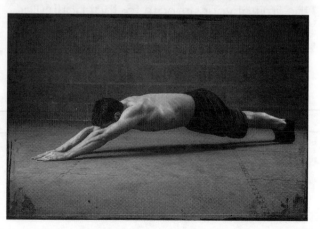

Arch

The arch is the first exercise we are going to look at in this chapter involving the muscles of the lower back to a large degree and, although it looks relatively simple, many people are caught out by its difficulty. It is an unusual position for most people to exert muscular force in, and this is probably why it can feel somewhat awkward at first. This movement is also the complete opposite to the dish position and exercise that we looked at earlier, and uses the opposing muscle groups.

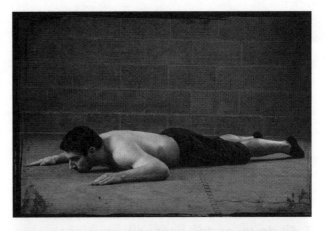

1. Lie face down on the ground with your arms bent at 90 degrees and held out to the sides.

2. Contract your back, butt, and leg muscles, and raise your torso off the floor as far as possible. Squeeze your shoulder blades together hard. You should be trying to make a shallow "U" shape, much as you were in the dish. Now hold this position for as long as possible.

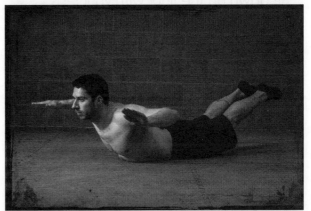

Teaching Points

Once the normal arch starts to become too easy, you can make the movement more challenging by extending your arms out in front of you in much the same way that the dish can be made more difficult by straightening the arms. This increases the workload on the muscles of the upper back, as well as moving more of the bodyweight away from the centre of gravity.

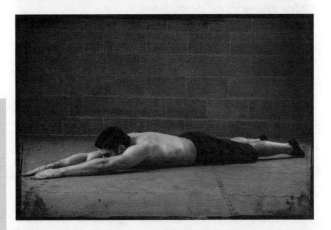

Start with 3 sets of 10-second holds, and then steadily increase from there.

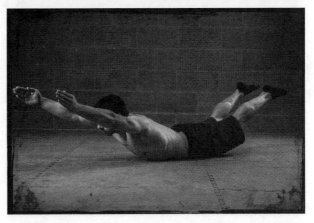

Rear Support

The rear support is another exercise taken from the gymnastic world that fits in with calisthenics perfectly. The rear support is essentially the opposite body position to the push-up, but because of the way the body is constructed, the rear support is much more difficult to hold than the familiar push-up position.

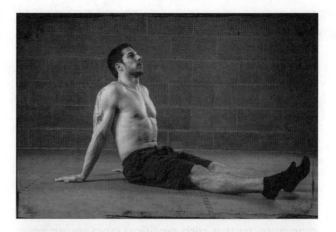

1. Sit down on the floor with your legs stretched out in front of you.

2. Place your hands by your hips with your fingers facing forwards. From here, push up hard with your arms and raise your hips as high as you can.

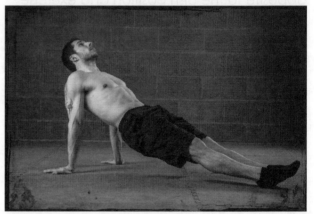

3. The aim is to get the shoulders, hips, knees, and ankles all in a straight line, with your chest and stomach facing the sky. Once you are in this position, hold it for as long as possible.

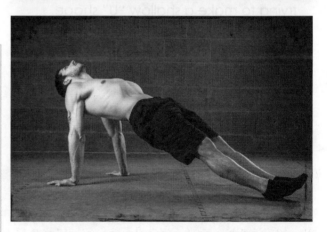

Teaching Points

Once the rear support becomes quite easy with your feet on the floor, you can start to elevate your feet by placing them on a platform or box, for example. This will put more of your bodyweight onto the target muscles and really requires you to contract your lower back hard.

You should start by trying to hold the position for 3 sets of 10 seconds, with no dropping of the hips. Steadily build your hold times from there.

Dragon Flag

This is the last of the floor core exercises. The dragon flag was made famous by Bruce Lee (which is why it is called the dragon flag), and requires very little equipment and provides a bit of variety from the other static core exercises in this chapter. You will need something solid and immovable to hold onto, such as the upright of a gym machine, or a bedpost. Experiment to find a suitable location. The dragon flag gives you an idea of what it is like for your core to support the entire weight of your lower body, and is a good supplemental exercise for use with the front lever.

As with the other more challenging movements in this book, I have broken the dragon flag down into manageable chunks to make it easier to progress. There are five stages:

1. Candlestick
2. Tucked dragon flag
3. Single-leg dragon flag
4. Negative dragon flag
5. Dragon flag

For all of these stages, it is advisable to use either a mat or something soft to pad the underside of the shoulders and back of the neck, as your entire bodyweight will be supported on them. I also often use a small platform or box to raise myself off the ground so that I feel a little less restricted by the floor.

You should also place the mat or box just short of your arms reach away from the bar or object that you will be holding so that your arms are slightly bent. This allows you to have some tension in the arms and also enables you to support the rest of your body adequately.

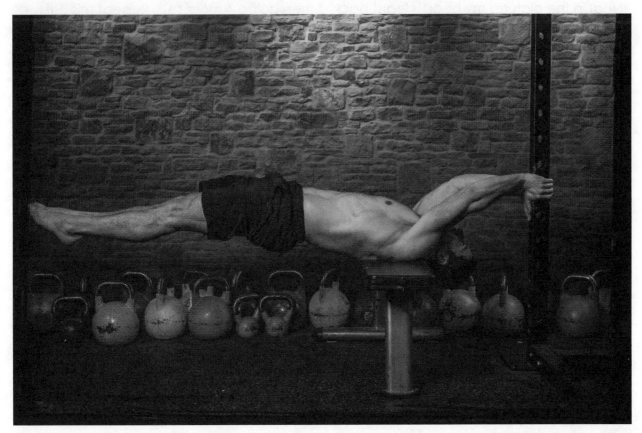

Candlestick

The first stage in learning the dragon flag is to be able to get your body into the top position, or what I have named the candlestick. This involves balancing on your shoulders and holding your legs vertically upright. It is quite daunting but the actual position is very safe.

1. Lie down and place your shoulders on the ground or a low box/platform.

2. Reach behind you and grab hold of the bar or the object you are using.

3. From here, tuck your knees into your chest and pull yourself up onto your shoulders until your torso becomes vertical. Now try and extend your legs fully until your knees are locked out. Point your toes to help align the body and generate muscular tension. Hold this position for as long as you can. Note that in the pictures my head is leant back slightly, which reduces the stress on the neck muscles.

Teaching Points

For this stage, all you should be concerned about is spending time in the position to get comfortable supporting yourself on your shoulders. I would recommend holding the candlestick position for as long as you can, then resting for 45 seconds or so, and then doing 4 more sets. Repeat this until you are confident in the position, and then move onto the next stage.

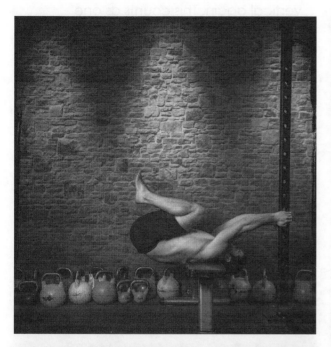

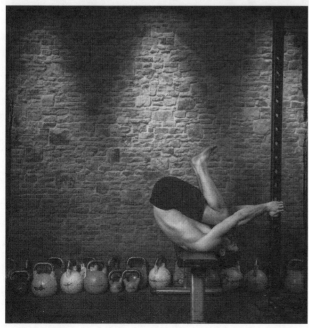

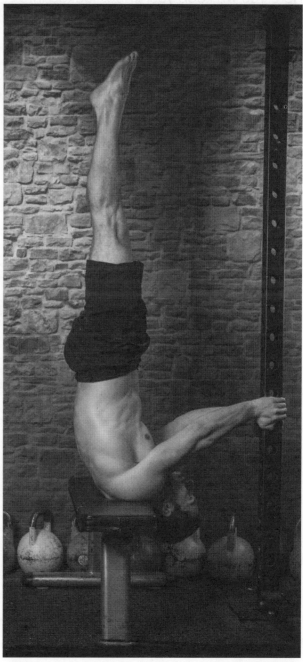

Tucked Dragon Flag

After you have perfected balancing on your shoulders you should start to work with the tucked version of the movement. Here you will keep your knees tucked into your chest and work with the complete movement.

1. Lay down with your arms over your head. Grasp the bar or object you are using with a strong grip.

2. From here, raise your legs and torso off the floor until your feet are pointing towards the ceiling. You should be balancing on your shoulders with your torso vertical and your knees tucked into your chest.

3. From this vertical position start to pivot around your shoulders and lower your entire body down towards the ground.

4. Keep going until your lower back nearly touches the ground, and then reverse the movement until your torso becomes vertical again. This counts as one repetition.

Teaching Points

You should be aiming to perform 4 sets of 5 to 6 repetitions. The dragon flag is meant to be a strength building movement, so the repetition range needs to be kept lower than some of the other core exercises within this chapter.

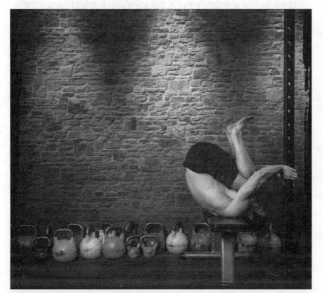

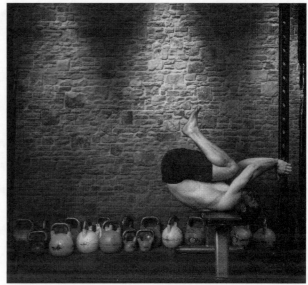

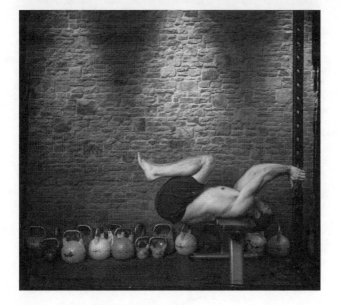

Single-Leg Dragon Flag

The single-leg dragon flag is halfway between the tucked variation and the full variation, and as such is the next stage in your dragon flag training.

1. Lay down with your arms over your head. Grasp the bar or object you are using with a strong grip.

2. From here, raise your legs and torso off the floor until you are positioned in a candlestick. Now tuck one leg tightly into your chest whilst keeping the other perfectly straight.

3. From this vertical position start to pivot around your shoulders and lower your entire body down towards the ground as slowly as possible. Keep a solid grip on the supporting bar or object that you are using. Do not allow your waist to bend at all during this movement. It is very important that all the movement occurs from your upper body.

4. Keep lowering yourself down until your entire body touches the ground. This counts as one repetition. Aim to perform 3 to 4 sets of 4 to 6 repetitions.

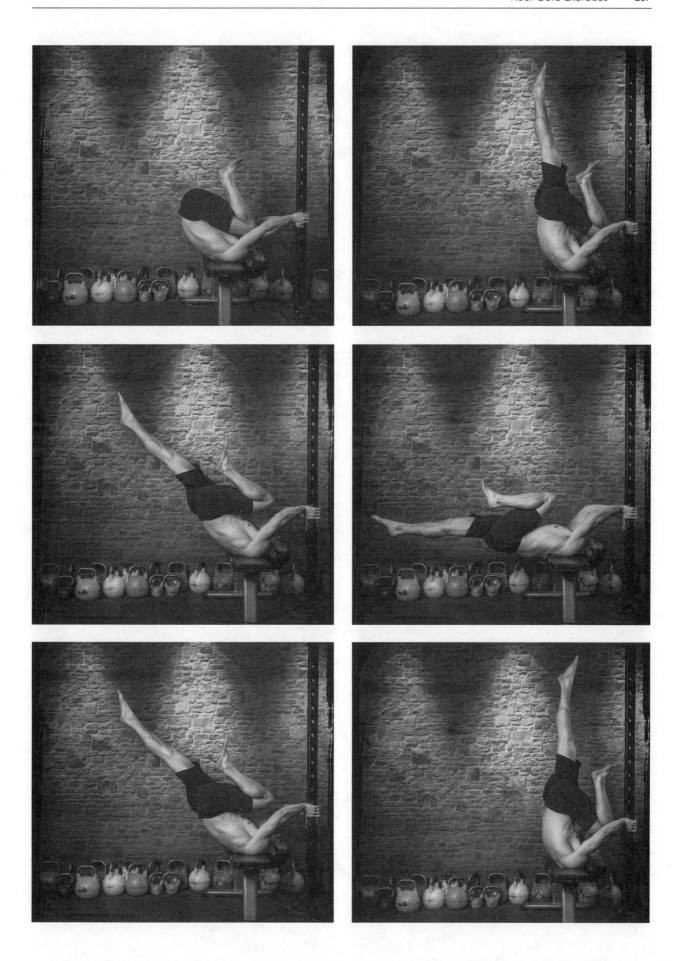

Negative Dragon Flag

Once you have worked hard enough with the tucked and the single-leg dragon flag, you can start to extend the legs out until your body is in a completely straight line. This stage has you working with negatives until you have built enough strength to perform the movement fully.

1. Lay down with your arms over your head. Grasp the bar or object you are using with a strong grip.

2. From here, raise your legs and torso off the floor until you are positioned in a candlestick. You should be balancing on your shoulders with your torso and legs completely vertical.

3. From this vertical position start to pivot around your shoulders and lower your entire body down towards the ground as slowly as possible. Keep a solid grip on the supporting bar or object that you are using. Do not allow your waist to bend at all during this movement. It is very important that all the movement occurs from your upper body.

4. Keep lowering yourself down until your entire body touches the ground. This counts as one repetition.

Teaching Points

As with other negative-type movements, such as the one-arm pull-up, the stresses and strains on the muscles, tendons and ligaments can be very high, so do not be concerned about performing lots of repetitions of this variation. I would recommend doing 5 sets of 2 to 3 repetitions, and if you go slowly enough in the negatives, then that should be sufficient to activate the muscles.

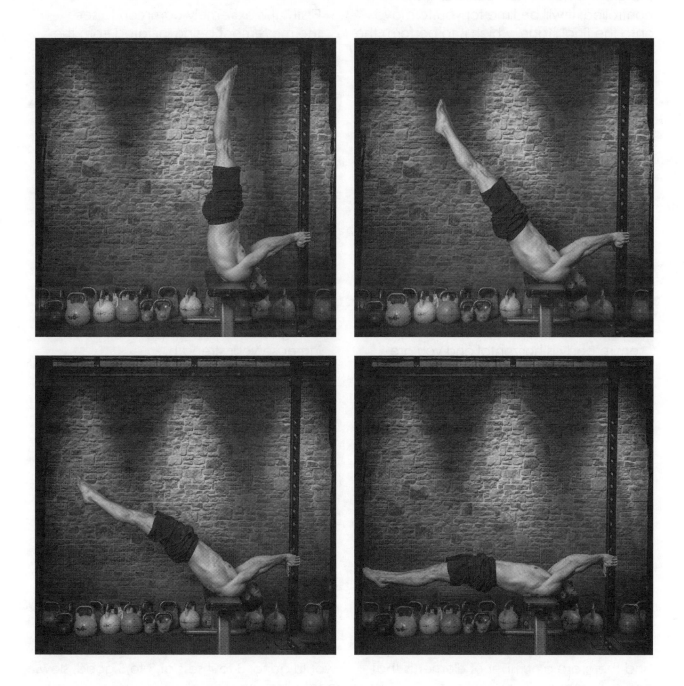

Dragon Flag

After you have spent enough time doing negatives, and the movement down to the ground has become slower and more controlled, it will be time for you to move onto the final stage, which is to perform the movement properly.

1. Lay down with your arms over your head and get into the candlestick position.

2. From this vertical position start to pivot around your shoulders and lower your entire body down towards the ground. Keep a solid grip on the supporting bar or object that you are using. Do not allow your waist to bend at all during this movement. It is very important that all the movement occurs from your upper body.

3. Keep lowering yourself down until your entire body is horizontal and you are a couple of inches from the ground. Now pull back up to the start position, keeping your body as straight as possible throughout the entire movement. You should try and prevent any bending at the waist. This counts as one repetition.

Teaching Points

The whole point of the dragon flag is to challenge the core to move the body whilst it is in a straight line. You must aim to pivot the body around the shoulders and keep the spine as straight as possible at all times. This is easier said than done however, and there are a number of elements that can go wrong:

- Firstly, it is extremely common to see the movement being initiated from the hips or the lower body. It is vital that the whole body moves as a single unit, with the toes, knees, hips, waist, and torso moving in a straight line with no kipping or what I call "worming", where one part of the body moves, and then another, etc.

- Secondly, you may have the situation where your core is strong enough to handle the movement but your upper body is not; in other words, you cannot support yourself properly on the bar or object that you are holding with your hands. To rectify this, spend more time doing upper body pulling exercises to increase your strength.

- Lastly, you may not be lowering yourself down until your body is horizontal. It is all too easy to think that your body is in the right position, but the reality may be very different. Performing the movement in front of a mirror, asking a training partner to help you, or even filming yourself, can be a great help here: using any of these methods will tell you immediately whether or not you are doing it correctly.

In terms of sets and repetitions, once again, this is a strength building exercise, so there is no need (and you may not be able) to perform lots of repetitions without tiring. I would go for 3 to 4 sets of 3 to 5 good, slow, controlled repetitions.

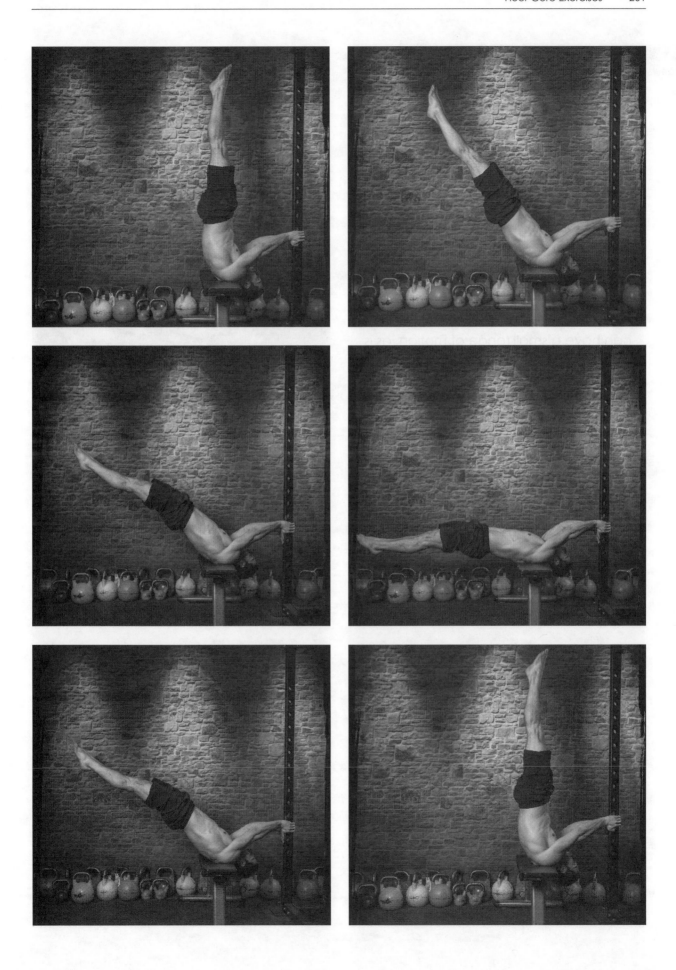

Dragon Flag Swimmers

We can make the dragon flag slightly more difficult by performing a swimming motion whilst holding the horizontal body position. These are very tough as your core muscles will have to not only hold the position but to move your legs as well.

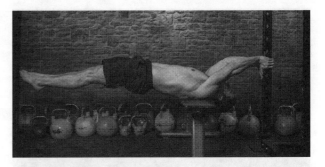

1. Get into a candlestick position and then lower down into a horizontal position.

2. Now move your legs up and down, as if you are swimming. Try and keep your knees locked as much as you can. You can have a small range of motion, as is shown in the pictures, or do slower wider swimming motions.

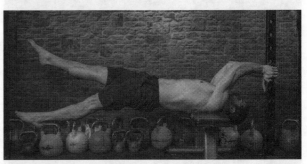

3. Keep doing this as long as you can and then either raise yourself back up into the candlestick position, or simply drop your feet down to the ground and rest. Try and perform as many repetitions as you can in 10 to 20 seconds.

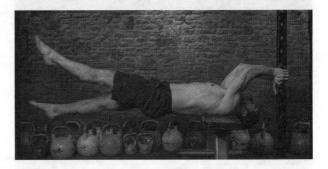

The second group of core exercises is those that can be performed on a pull-up bar. These exercises are particularly effective in building strength. This is because when the body is in a hanging position, the core is as stretched out as it can be, which makes contracting the muscles from that position more difficult, which in turn builds more strength. The movements in this chapter progress from the hanging knee raise, through the hanging leg raise, to the window wipers.

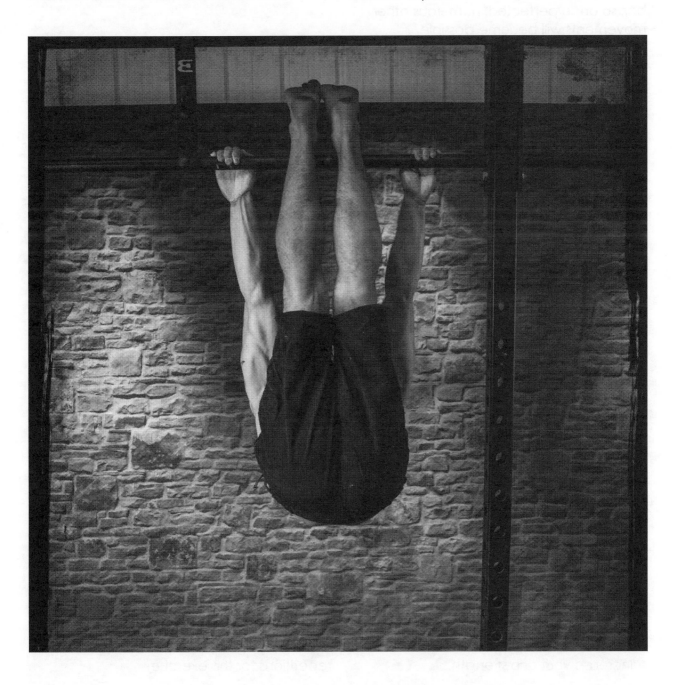

Hanging Knee Raise

The hanging knee raise is the first in this group of exercises to be performed on a pull-up bar. This means that as well as the core, your hands and grip strength will be worked as well. The hanging knee raise is also the gateway exercise to the core movements performed on the pull-up bar, so once perfected, numerous other movements will become possible.

1. Grab a pull-up bar with an overhand grip. Make sure that your arms are straight and your legs are hanging loosely.

2. Using your core muscles, raise your knees up as high as possible, tucking them into your chest if you can. In the pictures, you can see the widest range of motion that is possible, so just keep working towards this. Try to eliminate any swing by pulling down slightly with your arms.

3. Lower your legs down to the start position. This counts as one repetition.

Teaching Points

There are a few common difficulties with both the hanging knee raise and the hanging leg raise (see next exercise):

- Firstly, most people have a problem with their grip, in that they cannot hold onto the bar long enough to start working the core muscles. To remedy this, we can simply hang from a pull-up bar for a set amount of time. As your grip strength increases, you will be able to perform hanging knee raises much more easily. Your other training, e.g. pull-ups, will also increase your grip strength.

- Secondly, there is the issue of not having enough core strength to actually lift up your knees. To address this, simply raise up your knees as far as you can, and with practice, as with all of the other exercises, your strength will increase and the movement will become easier.

- Thirdly, there is the issue of not being able to control your swing, or of using too much momentum to raise the knees. To control excessive swinging you will need to pull down slightly with your arms. This should feel very similar to the vertical pulls that we looked at in the front lever section. This should help to lean back the body slightly, which will eliminate any swing that may occur.

- Finally, you must try and use as little momentum to raise the knees as possible. This may feel tempting, especially in the early stages where you are struggling to perform the movement properly, but it will inhibit your progress in the later stages, and is a bad habit to get into.

Start by trying to perform 3 or 4 sets of 8 repetitions for this exercise.

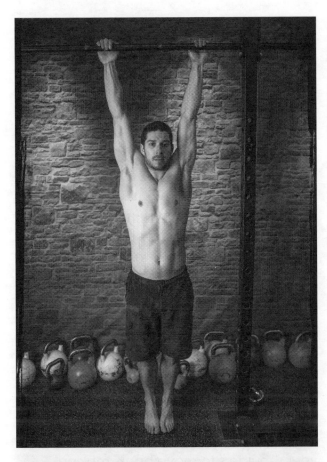
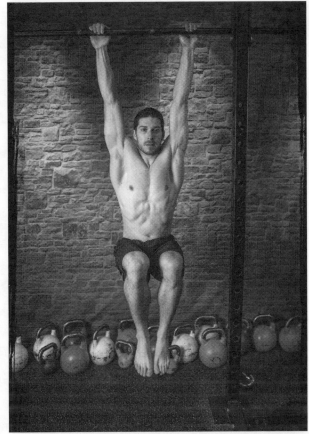
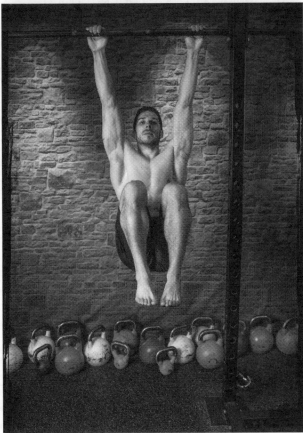
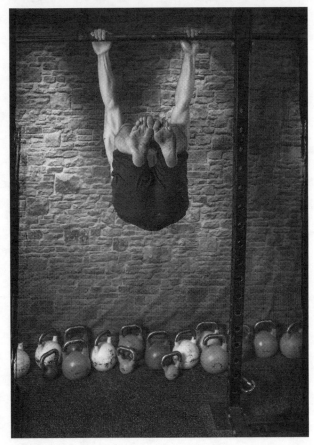

Hanging Leg Raise

Once you have mastered the hanging knee raise, and you can comfortably tuck your knees all the way up to your chest, it is time to move onto the hanging leg raise. The ultimate aim of this exercise is to hang from a bar, and with straight legs, raise them up until your toes reach your hands. This movement requires both a strong core and flexibility.

1. Grasp a pull-up bar with an overhand grip and hang with your arms completely straight.

2. Pull down slightly with your arms to minimise the momentum. From here, start to raise your legs up as high as you can whilst keeping your knees locked out.

3. Keep raising your legs until your feet reach your hands.

4. Lower your legs slowly until they reach the start position. This counts as one repetition.

Teaching Points

At first you may not have the strength to raise your legs all the way to your hands. If this is the case, just raise them as far as you can. Your strength will increase over time, and eventually you will be able to raise your legs to your hands.

If you find that you cannot eliminate the momentum, or you find that you are swinging excessively when performing the exercise, have someone push on the back of your shoulders. This will stop you from being able to pull down, which allows your shoulders to move back, making the exercise easier. You should be aiming to perform at least 4 sets of 8 repetitions eventually.

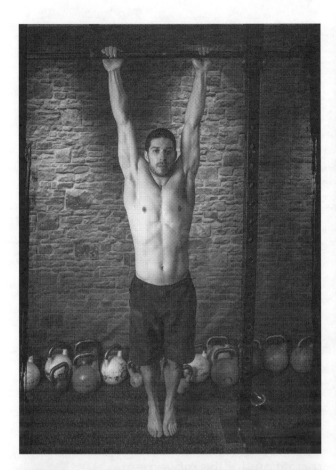

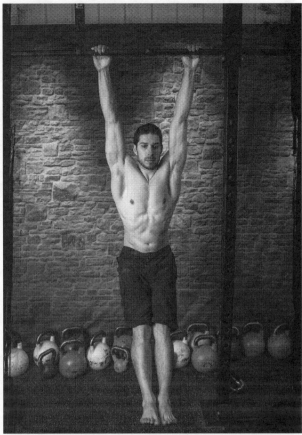

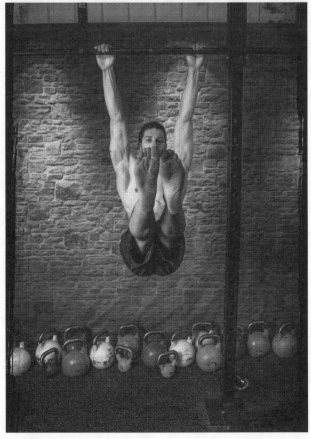

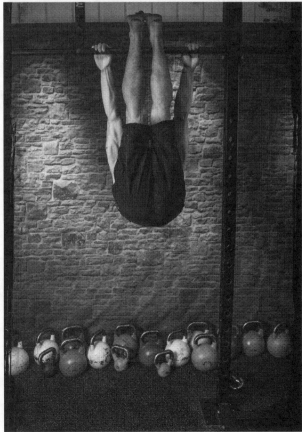

Window Wipers

Window wipers are an awesome variation on the hanging leg raise and require a huge amount of abdominal strength. Before you attempt this movement you should make sure that you can perform a proper full hanging leg raise and be able to get your toes to the bar quite easily.

1. Hang from a pull-up bar with an overhand grip. Raise your toes up to the bar, keeping your legs as straight as you can.

2. From here, move your legs over to one side, aiming to keep your arms as straight as possible. Keep the toes in line with the pull-up bar at all times.

3. Keep moving your legs over as far as your flexibility will allow. Then move them over to the opposite side and repeat the movement.

Teaching Points

One of the main problems that people run into when trying to perform window wipers is that they cannot keep their legs close enough to the bar to complete the movement. To practice this, simply perform a hanging leg raise and hold your feet at the top of the position for as long as you can.

Try and perform 3 or 4 sets of at least 6 repetitions for this movement.

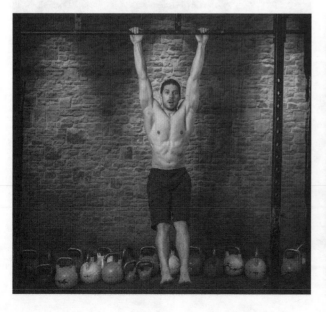

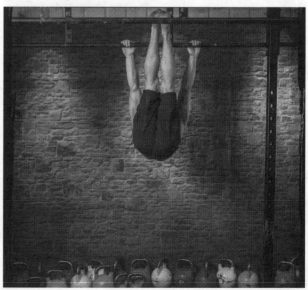

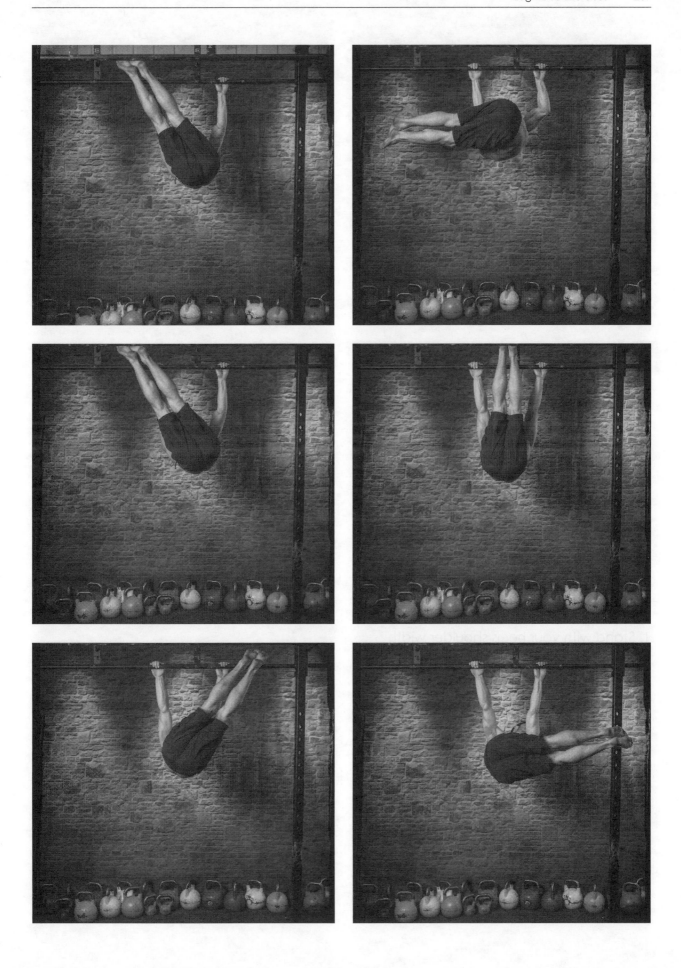

As stated in Chapter 1, traditionally the lower body has not been the most widely trained body part for many calisthenic enthusiasts over the years, but hopefully I can help to change that view. In fact, in some similar books on bodyweight training, the lower body is not even mentioned, with the emphasis on the development of the upper body and core. I really disagree with this, as, in my opinion, calisthenics should be about developing a complete physique that is capable of performing the widest range of movement possible in the greatest number of situations. This is why the lower body must be included.

In this chapter I have chosen to include exercises that develop both pure strength and power. It is all very well building huge amounts of strength, but that strength must be put to good use, e.g. jumping long distances or jumping onto a high platform.

Squat

The squat is one of the most basic and most fundamental of human movements. As Mark Rippetoe observes in his book, *Starting Strength*, it involves a vital part of athletic preparation, i.e. hip drive. Hip drive consists of two factors: knee and hip extension, which means that the angles of both these joints increase. Knee extension involves the muscles from the quads, or the front of the thigh, and hip extension uses three muscle groups: the glutes, hamstrings, and adductors.

1. Stand with your heels shoulder width apart and your hands folded across your chest or held out in front of you. Your toes should be pointed out at around 30 degrees, although this will differ slightly depending on your physiology and flexibility.

2. Bend at the knees, keeping your back as straight as possible and your eyes looking forwards. Push your hips back and down at the same time. As you descend, push your knees out and let your hips drop between the gap in your knees. Also make sure that your feet stay as flat as possible, with no part of the sole coming off the floor at any time.

3. Keep squatting down as low as you physically can. As your strength, mobility and flexibility increase, you should be able to squat lower and lower. In the pictures opposite, you can see that I have good mobility and my hips are much lower than my knees. This may take you some time to achieve, but persevere and you will reach your goal.

4. From this bottom position, drive the hips up until you reach the start position. This counts as one repetition.

Teaching Points

The squat is quite a complex movement, with a lot of interplay between muscles and joints and is actually quite easy to perform incorrectly. Squats also require a surprising degree of flexibility. If you cannot get your hip joint low enough to become

44444444444444444

level with your knee joint, then just squat down as low as you can. As your strength and flexibility increases with time, you will be able to descend increasingly lower. In addition, the squat is also one of the fundamental five movements discussed previously. The target is to be able to do 25 perfect repetitions, so I would recommend trying 3 to 4 sets of 10 and then build from there.

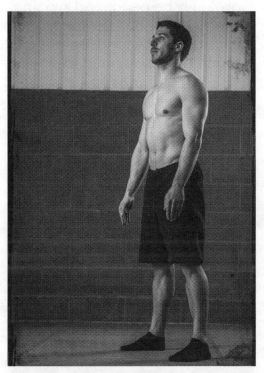
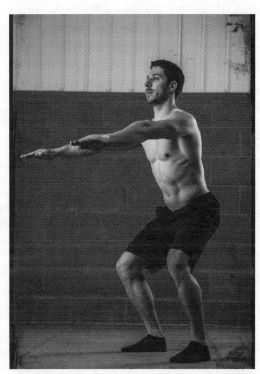
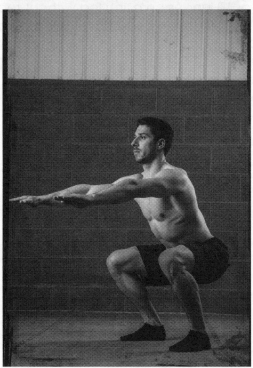
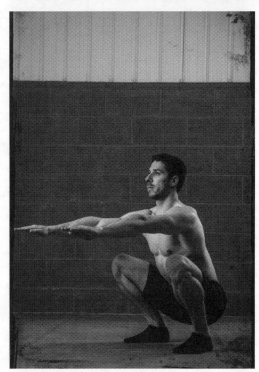

Lunge

Whilst squats are good for developing mobility and strength in a stationary position, we can use lunges to develop power and strength in a more natural running gait. You can either concentrate on one leg at a time or alternate between left and right. In my experience, most people find the lunge marginally more challenging than the squat as more pressure is placed on one leg with each movement.

1. Stand with your feet shoulder width apart and your hands by your sides.

2. Step forwards with one leg as if you were taking a big stride. Make sure that the heel hits the ground first followed by the rest of the foot.

3. From this position bend both legs until your rear knee nearly touches the ground. Try and keep your torso as upright as possible throughout the entire movement.

4. From this bottom position you can either push down hard with the front foot and return back to the standing position, or you can push off hard with the rear leg and step forwards. The first method can obviously be performed in a small area, as you are essentially standing in one spot, but the second requires a little bit of space as you will need to move forwards.

5. Make sure that you also use both legs equally to avoid developing any strength imbalances.

Teaching Points

As with many of the other exercises, if you cannot drop your knee to the floor then just work with a reduced range of motion. As your strength builds you will be able to drop lower and lower, which acts to stretch out the muscles in the lower body and the movement should become more effective. You should be able to perform 3 or 4 sets of 10 lunges on each leg without too much trouble, even if you have only just started training.

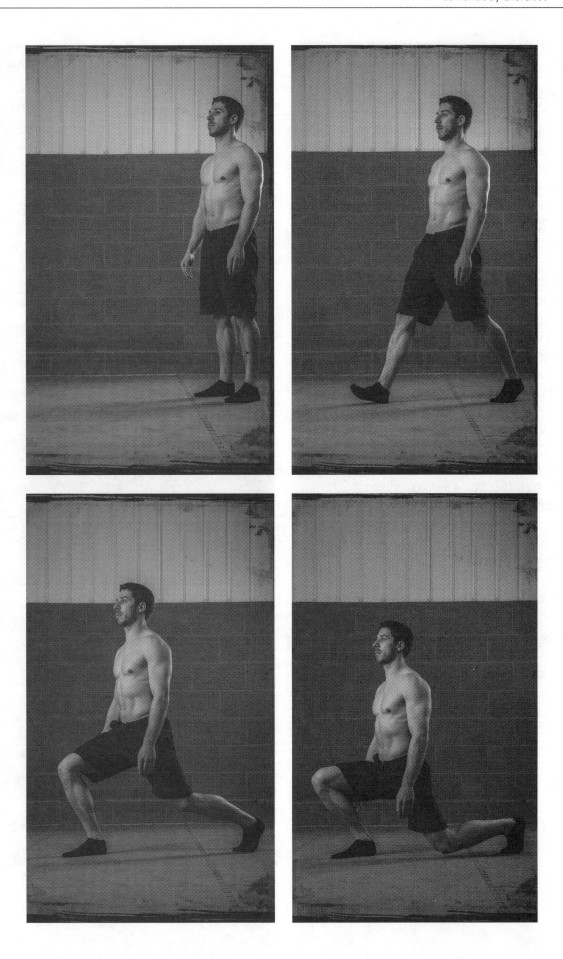

Bridge

The bridge is another exercise that we can use to target the rear of the lower body. It is a static exercise, which means that there is no movement involved and that the muscles will have to contract for a given amount of time. This is similar in principle to the rear support that we looked at on page 250, apart from the bridge does not require the use of the upper body.

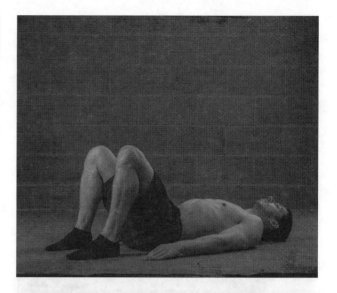

1. Lie on your back with your feet flat on the floor, and your knees at 90 degrees.

2. Keeping your shoulders pressed firmly into the ground, raise your hips up as high as possible. Aim to get your knees, hips, and shoulders into a straight line. Note that the feet stay flat and the head is resting on the floor.

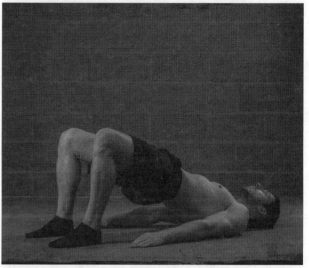

3. Now hold this position for as long as you can: aim for 3 or 4 sets of at least 20 seconds.

Teaching Points

To make this movement more difficult, you can simply perform it with only one leg on the ground and the other sticking up into the air. This puts added stress not only on the glutes and the hamstrings but also the core, as it is forced to fight the twisting motion of the body.

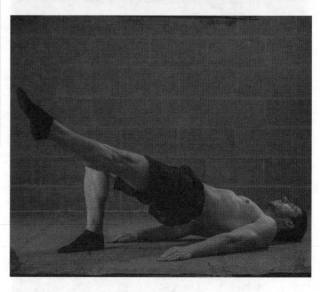

Calf Raise

The calves are involved in squats, lunges and all lower body movements, but we can use a specific exercise to work them in isolation. This is useful if you feel that the other lower body exercises do not work them enough, or if you feel that your calf development is lacking.

1. Stand with your feet shoulder width apart.

2. From here, contract your calf muscles hard and raise yourself up onto your toes.

3. Then lower back down to the start position. This counts as one repetition.

Teaching Points

To increase the resistance, you can add weight to the movement by holding a weight in each hand. Dumbbells or kettlebells are excellent for this and can be found in many different weights in any gym. You should try to perform 3 to 4 sets of 10 repetitions. Make sure that you perform the movement as slowly as possible.

You can also perform the calf raise in a crouching position, which adds a little bit of a balance challenge.

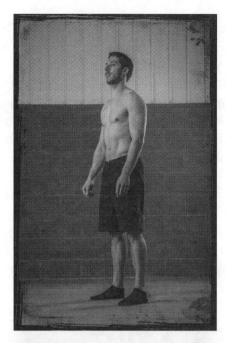

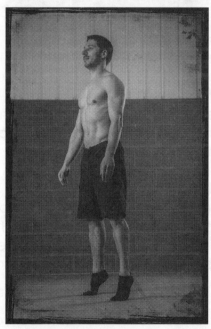

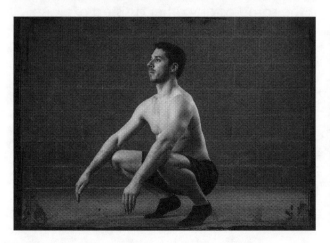

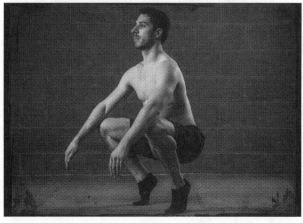

Single-Leg Squat

Once you have perfected the squat you can start training for the single-leg squat (or SLS), a true, unassisted squat using a single leg. It requires a huge amount of leg strength, not to mention balance, muscle control, and active flexibility.

Like the one-arm push-up and the one-arm pull-up, the single-leg squat is a unilateral exercise, and as such, builds huge amounts of strength and athletic proficiency. I have broken the movement down into four different stages:

1. Assisted single-leg squat
2. Single-leg box squat
3. Single-leg squat
4. Weighted single-leg squat

Assisted Single-Leg Squat

To start your SLS training, you need to be able to assist yourself with your arms. There are a number of ways that this can be done, from using a suspension trainer, to a doorframe, to a random gym machine. All that is needed is simply something that you can hold onto that is sturdy enough for you to pull on.

1. Assume a one-footed stance. Grab the apparatus you are using with both hands, making sure that you have a secure hold. In the picture I am holding onto a squat rack frame, but anything sturdy will do.

2. Extend your free leg and lock out your knee. From here, start to bend your leg and lower yourself down to the ground.

3. Use your arms to support yourself and aid your balance. Keep lowering until you can go no further: your depth will depend on a number of factors, including your strength, flexibility, and mobility.

4. From the bottom position, push up hard with your leg until you reach the standing position again. Use your arms as much as you need to assist you in standing up again. This counts as one repetition.

Teaching Points

Working with the assisted single-leg squat is the same as any other assisted exercise. As you become stronger, you can simply reduce the amount of assistance that you are using and move more of the exercise onto the target muscles.

Try and perform 3 to 4 sets of 5 repetitions on each leg, and then do more as your strength increases.

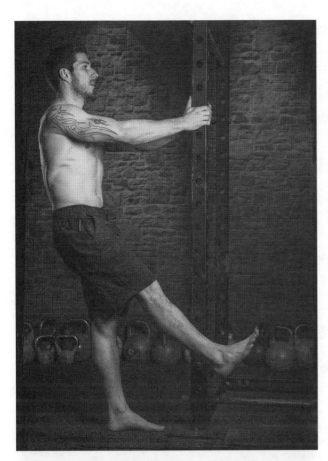

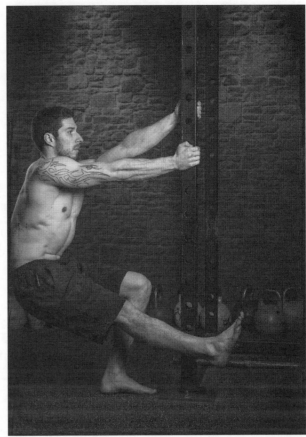

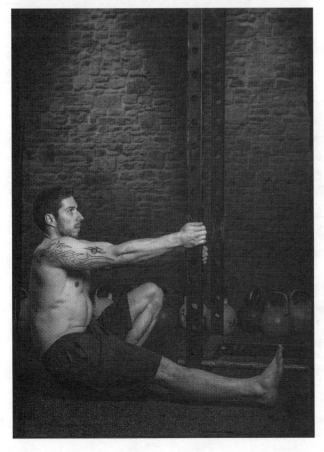

Single-Leg Box Squat

The second stage in learning the single-leg squat is to use a platform or similar to stand on that will allow your free leg to dangle down instead of being held up. This makes the movement easier and allows you to experiment with the exercise.

1. Assume a one-footed stance on your box. Hold your arms out in front of you to aid your balance.

2. Keeping your free leg straight and extended, start to bend your knee and stick your hips back.

3. Keep bending your knee as far as you can. Once you are sitting down fully, keep the tension on the legs.

4. From here, push up hard until you reach the start position. This counts as one repetition.

Teaching Points

As with many of the other exercises, to progress with the SLS you need to make the movement more manageable. To do this, simply bend your knee only a small amount, which will allow you to work with a reduced range of motion. As you become stronger, squat down lower.

To start with, try and perform 3 to 4 sets of 5 repetitions on each leg, and increase the number as your strength increases.

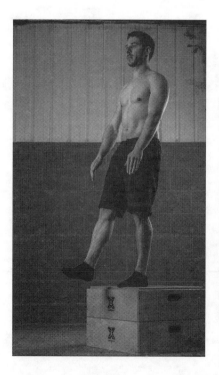
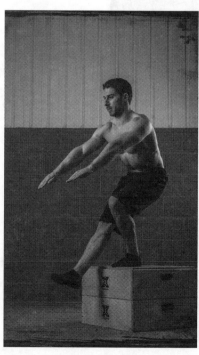
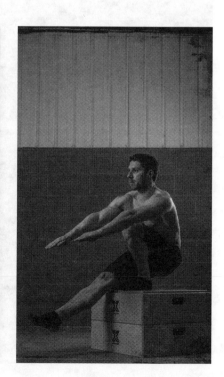

Single-Leg Squat

Once you have spent enough time with the two variations presented so far, you will be ready to start working on the full version. The full single-leg squat will require more flexibility and mobility than the other two variations, and it will probably take you some time to perfect the movement.

1. Stand on one leg with the other leg held as horizontal as possible.

2. Squat down on the grounded leg, keeping your heel on the floor. Putting your arms out in front of you can help with balance.

3. Once you reach the bottom of the movement, push back up until you return to the start position. This counts as one repetition.

Teaching Points

The single-leg squat is a very challenging exercise, but fortunately we can use a simple technique we looked at earlier to help. The best way to train the single-leg squat is by using negatives. This will involve doing the negative portion of the squat, and then rolling backwards onto your back to recover, or placing your other foot down on the ground and standing up with two legs.

Another technique that we can use is to place the working leg on a sloped platform. This will enable you to increase your range of motion even if you have low mobility or flexibility.

Once you reach this stage, try and perform 3 to 4 sets of 5 repetitions on each leg, and only increase this to a maximum of 8 to 10 repetitions before moving onto the weighted version, shown next.

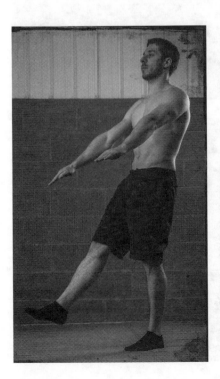
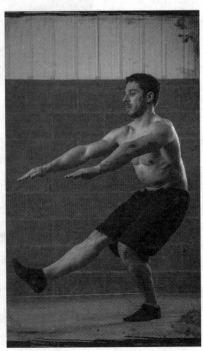
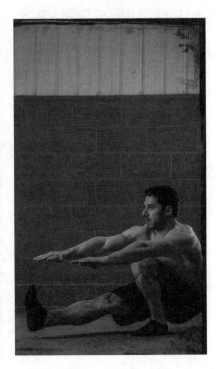

Weighted Single-Leg Squat

Once you have become fairly proficient with the normal single-leg squat, you can add some weight to the exercise to make it a little more challenging. This can be achieved in a variety of ways but the best is probably to use a dumbbell. These can be found in a variety of weights in any commercial gym. Ironically, some people actually find the weighted version of this movement slightly easier, as the weight can act to help your balance.

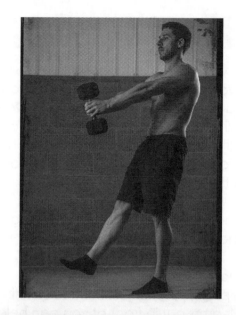

1. Grasp the weight you are using in both hands and hold it out at arm's length.

2. Stand on one leg and extend the other out in front of you.

3. From here, squat down on one leg as far as possible, aiming to get your hamstrings to touch your calf. Make sure that your free leg remains straight.

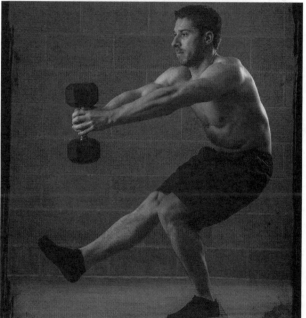

4. To help you balance, use the weight that you are holding in your hands as a counterbalance. For example, if you feel yourself falling over backwards, move the weight further forwards. If you find yourself falling forwards, bring the weight closer to your torso.

5. From the bottom push down hard with your leg until you return to a standing position. This counts as one repetition.

Teaching Points

It goes without saying that as you become stronger and more proficient you should add more weight. Keep progressing like this as long as you need to. Again, you should try and hit at least 3 sets of 5 repetitions on each leg, for 3 to 4 sets.

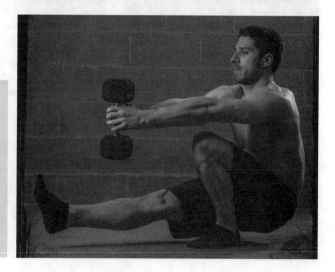

Hamstring Curl

Traditionally the hamstrings have been trained using the squat and lunge, as the quads work together with them to balance forces on each side of the knee. In recent years it has been in vogue to use hamstring curl machines to isolate the muscle and apply extra resistance. This is adequate for most people, but if we are serious about developing extreme strength, then we need a better exercise. The hamstring curl is effectively a bodyweight biceps curl using the hamstrings. It is an extremely tough movement that can take a long time to master, but once you can perform a few perfect repetitions, your hamstrings will be absolutely bulletproof.

In terms of equipment and apparatus required for this movement, you will need a place where you can kneel down with a vertical torso and something to secure your ankles, such as the underside of a squat rack, a dumbbell, or even a training partner. Experiment until you find a suitable location. It is also recommended that you pad the knees to protect the knee joint. Below is a picture that shows how to do this.

As this is such a challenging movement, we will break it down into manageable stages to make progression easier and injury less likely. These are:

1. Piked hamstring curl
2. Assisted hamstring curl
3. Negative hamstring curl
4. Hamstring curl

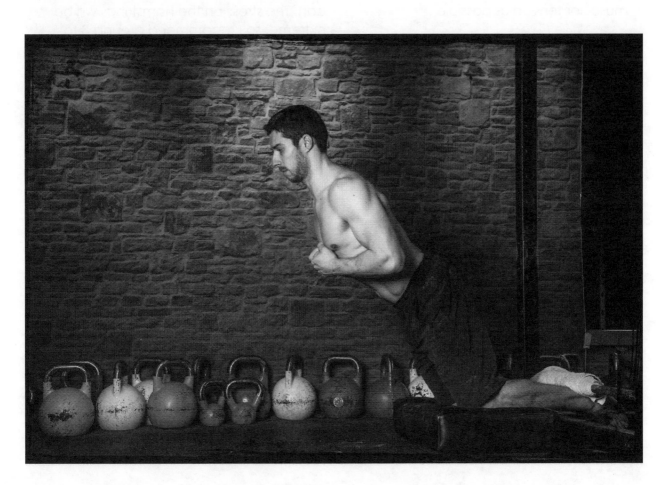

Piked Hamstring Curl

The initial stage in learning this movement is to attempt to reduce the load on the hamstrings whilst still performing the exercise. To do this we can simply pike, or bend, at the hips. This lessens the amount of stress on the hamstrings and glutes, and also reduces the range of motion of the movement.

1. Secure your ankles and pad the underside of your knees.

2. Bend forwards at the hips, keeping the thighs as vertical as possible: the greater the bend, the easier the movement.

3. Keeping the angle at the hips consistent, start to lower yourself down towards the ground. Contract all of your muscles as hard as you can to generate as much muscular tension as possible.

4. As soon as you touch the ground with the upper body (or get close to touching it), curl yourself back up to the start position. This counts as one repetition.

Teaching Points

As you progress with the piked hamstring curl, you should simply reduce the bend in the hips. This will make the movement more difficult to perform. On the other end of the scale, if you need to make the exercise easier, then just increase the bend in the hips.

For sets and repetitions, it is advisable to keep the number of each as low as you can. The stress on the hamstrings will be extreme, so I recommend around 3 to 4 sets of 3 to 5 repetitions to start with. I would not go any higher as this is meant to be a strength building exercise and not a muscular endurance one.

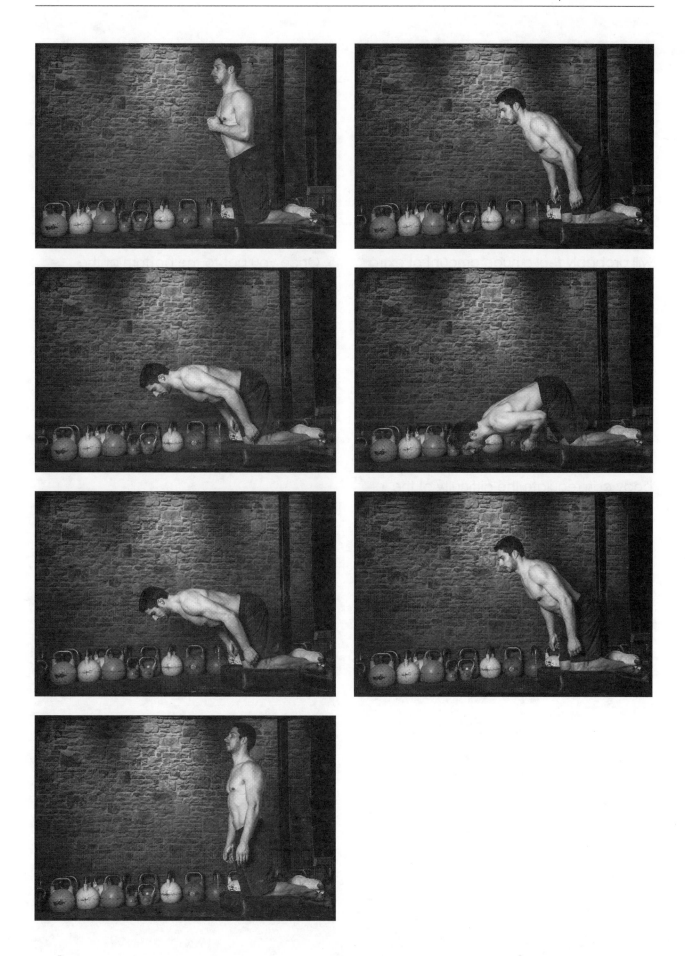

Assisted Hamstring Curl

Once you can perform a number of good repetitions with the hips in a piked position, you can start extending the hips and attempting the full movement. The likelihood is that you will still be too weak to execute a solid repetition, so in this stage we will use the upper body to assist with the exercise, and try to eliminate the pike or bend in the hips completely. You will probably feel a huge amount of extra tension and stress in the lower back as a result of this, but this is to be expected as the leverage is decreased to very low levels.

In this movement you will also be using the upper body to assist with the exercise. There are a number of ways of doing this but one of the simplest is to use either a box, a bar or raised platform on which to place the hands. This way your upper body can regulate the difficulty of the movement through the entirety of the exercise. In this example I have used a simple bar to assist.

1. Secure your ankles and pad the underside of your knees.

2. Ensure that your hips are completely open, and that the shoulders, hips, and knees form a straight line.

3. Place your hands on the object that you are using and start to lower yourself down towards the ground. Keep as much tension throughout the body as possible.

4. As you descend use your hands and upper body to reduce the amount of stress on the hamstrings.

5. Once you get to the bottom of the movement, use your upper body to push hard against the object and contract your hamstrings, glutes, and lower back to return to the start position. This counts as one repetition.

Teaching Points

Again, as with the other methods of this type, you can reduce the assistance from the upper body as your strength increases. Sets and repetitions should be the same as the previous variation, being 3 to 4 sets of 3 to 5 repetitions at the most.

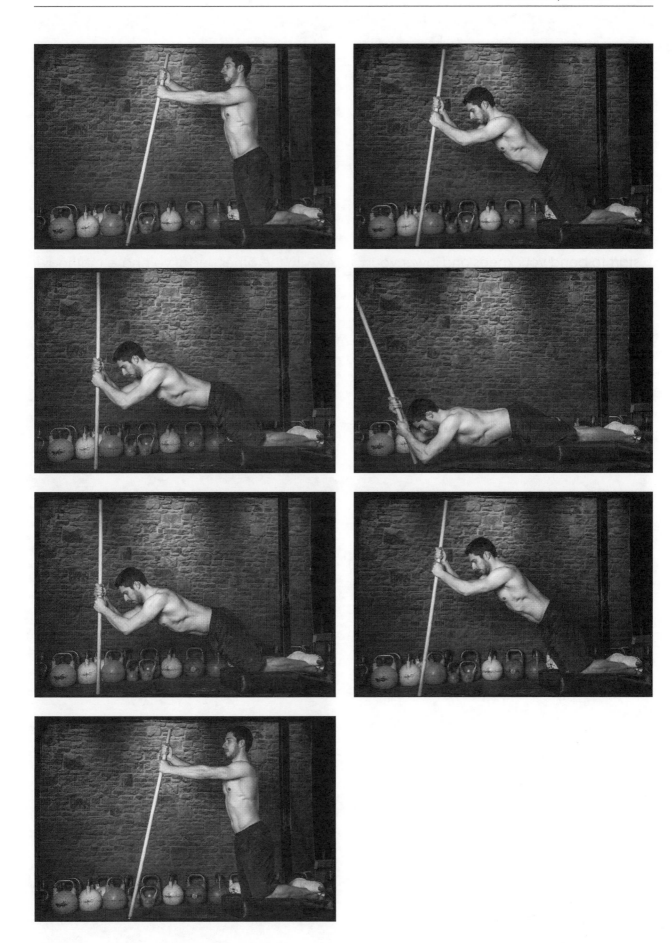

Negative Hamstring Curl

The third stage in learning the hamstring curl is the negative variation. This is the final stage before working on the proper movement.

1. Secure your ankles and pad the underside of your knees.

2. Keeping your torso as straight as possible, start to bend your knees and lower your body down to the ground. Try and make this movement as slow as possible.

3. Clench your fists and attempt to generate as much muscular tension as you can.

4. As soon as your torso reaches the ground, place your hands on the floor and push yourself back up to the start position. This counts as one repetition.

Teaching Points

As with the other negative phase methods, you should be looking to slow the movement down as you become stronger. You can also reduce the amount of help the upper body gives you to return to the start position.

Sets and repetitions should be slightly reduced compared to the previous variation, as the stress on the target muscles is much more extreme. Try 3 to 4 sets of 1 to 3 repetitions at the most.

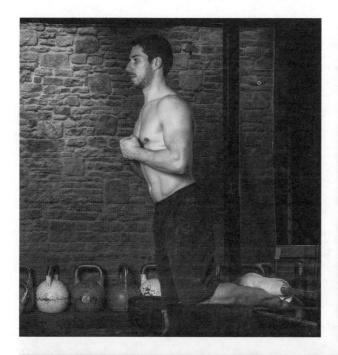
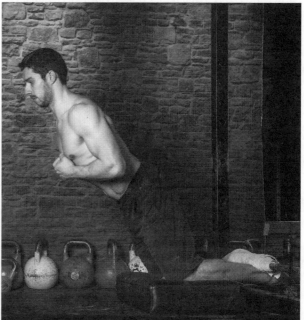
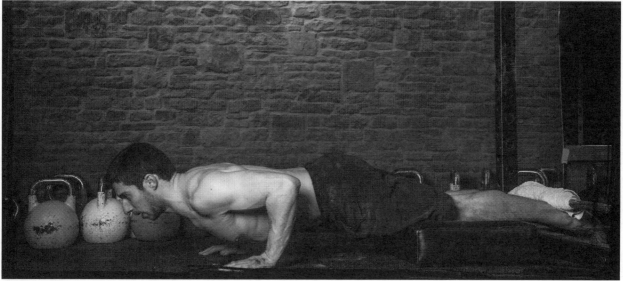

Hamstring Curl

Once you have spent some time with the negative variation, then all that remains is to perform the movement without the help of the upper body. This is an immensely difficult movement, so take your time and only progress when you feel that you are ready.

1. Secure your ankles and pad the underside of your knees.

2. Put your arms across your chest and keep your body straight.

3. Lower down, pivoting from your knees until your torso nearly touches the floor. Do not allow your hips to bend. Note in the pictures that the lower back remains straight at all times.

4. From here, contract hard with your hamstrings, glutes and lower back to return to the upright position. This counts as one repetition.

Teaching Points

In terms of sets and repetitions, I would simply do what you can. The chances are that you will struggle massively to achieve double figures, so just concentrate on the quality of the movement above all else. You should be aiming to do 3 sets of 3 to 5 repetitions eventually.

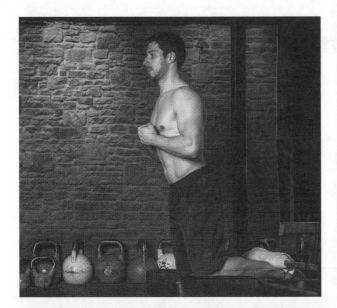

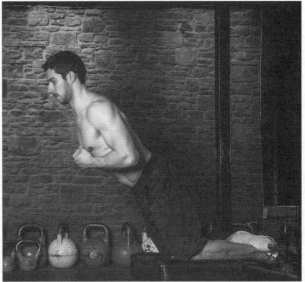

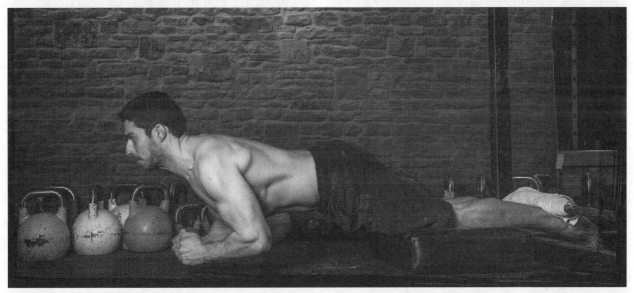

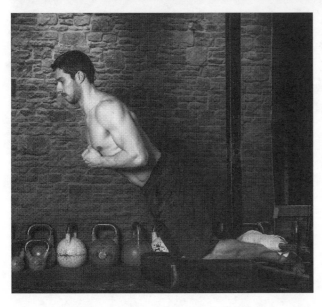

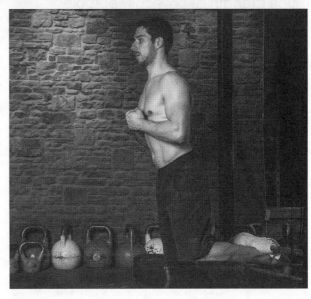

Although conditioning would not traditionally be included in many calisthenic workouts, I think that it deserves a place in most people's training regime. Conditioning can be defined as the body's ability to do an immense amount of work in a short period of time.

There are two types of cardiovascular exercise that we can use to train our lungs and cardiovascular system:

1. Aerobic exercise is physical activity in which energy is produced with the aid of oxygen. Walking and light running are examples of this type of exercise.

2. Anaerobic exercise is more intense physical activity where energy is produced without the aid of oxygen. This form of exercise is extremely intense and tiring, and really takes a lot of mental power and determination to smash through. A good example would be the 100 meters sprint.

Although this is not a book about conditioning, more about building as much strength as physically possible using calisthenic training, being fit and conditioned makes your workouts easier, enabling you to keep going for longer, which can only lead to better results in a shorter period of time. As such, do not feel that you have to perform burpees or sprints every time you train. Once every one or two weeks should be enough, and you can leave them out altogether if you so wish.

Star Jumps

Star jumps are a key exercise of militaries around the world. They are straightforward to perform, can be made more difficult in a number of ways, and can also act as a good warm-up exercise.

1. Stand with your feet together and your arms by your sides.

2. Jump up into the air, and move your feet and arms out to the side as you do so.

3. Keep moving the feet and arms out until you land on the ground again, by which point your feet will be widely spaced apart and your arms will be raised above your head.

4. From this position, jump again and bring your feet back to the centre and your arms back down towards your sides. This counts as one repetition.

Teaching Points

Try and perform 3 sets of 20 repetitions as fast as you can. You can also try and do as many repetitions in a specific time period as possible. For example, see how many repetitions you can do in 3 sets of 60 seconds.

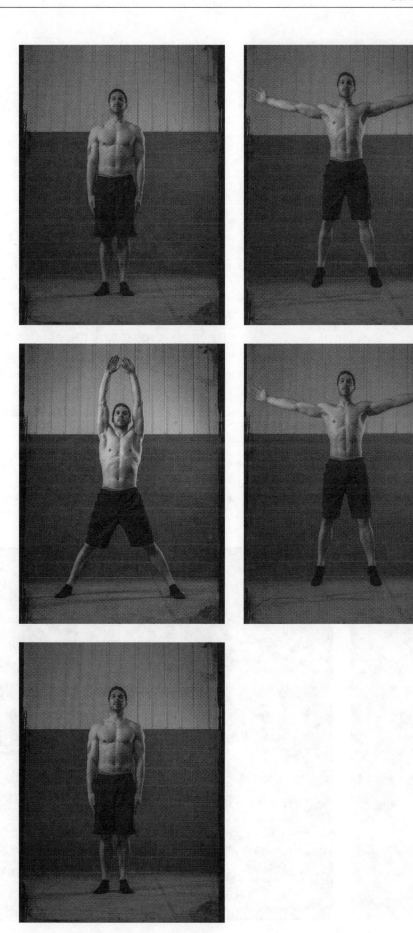

Jumping Squat

Normal bodyweight squats are awesome for developing lower body strength, and we can use a variation of them for our conditioning as well. Jump squats are exactly what they sound like: squats where you jump at the top of each repetition.

1. Stand with your feet shoulder width apart and your knees slightly bent.

2. Squat down as low as you can, using the same technique as for the normal bodyweight squat.

3. From this bottom position push up hard with the legs and jump as high as you can into the air.

4. As you land, bend your knees to absorb the shock and continue with the exercise.

Teaching Points

In terms of sets and repetitions, try and do the same as for the star jumps; 3 sets of 20 repetitions as fast as you can. You can also try and do as many repetitions in a specific time period as possible. For example, see how many repetitions you can achieve in 3 sets of 60 seconds.

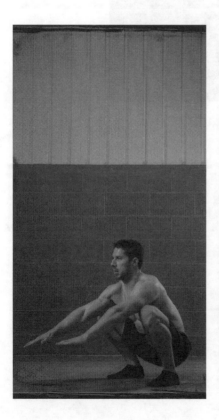
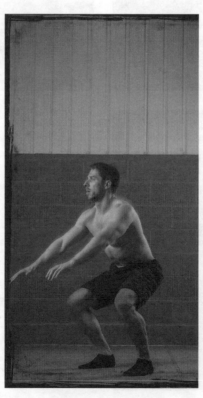
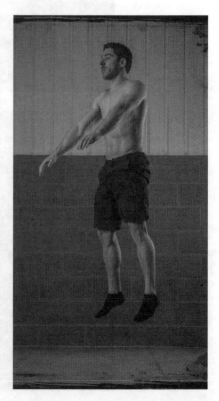

Jumping Lunge

As with the normal bodyweight squats, lunges can also be used as an excellent conditioning exercise. They are more challenging than jumping squats, as the front leg will take the brunt of the force and impact as you take off and land. They can be made easier by not dipping as low on each repetition, but this will also diminish your results.

1. Stand with your feet in the extended lunge position.

2. Drop down until your rear knee is nearly touching the ground. At this point your torso should be upright and both of your knees should be at around 90 degrees.

3. From here, push up hard with both of your legs and jump into the air as high as you can.

4. In midair, switch your legs around so that your front leg moves to the rear position and the back leg moves to the front position.

5. Bend your knees to absorb the impact when you land, and then repeat for the desired number of repetitions.

Teaching Points

As jumping lunges are more challenging than jumping squats, you will want to perform slightly fewer of them. Try 3 sets of 8 repetitions on each leg, and then build up from there. You can of course do sets for specific amounts of time, such as 3 sets of 40 seconds, and so on.

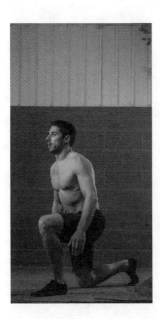
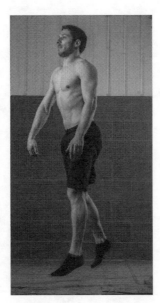
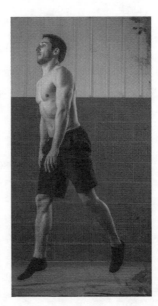
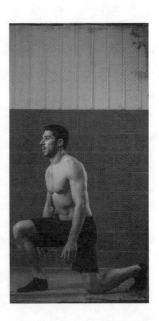

Squat Thrust

Squat thrusts are a little more challenging than the exercises we have looked at so far, and will really help to increase your heart rate. The squat thrust is also the first part of the burpee, which we will look at shortly, and so can be used by those of you looking for an easier exercise to get started with. They also require a little bit more mobility than the other conditioning exercises that have been presented so far.

1. Crouch down and place your hands flat on the floor. This is the start and finish position. From here, jump your feet into the air and extend your legs out backwards until you land in the top of a push-up position.

2. From here, jump your feet into the air and return them to the crouched position. This counts as one repetition.

Teaching Points

Try and perform 3 sets of 20 repetitions as fast as you can. You can also try and do as many repetitions in a specific time period as possible. For example, see how many repetitions you can achieve in 3 sets of 60 seconds.

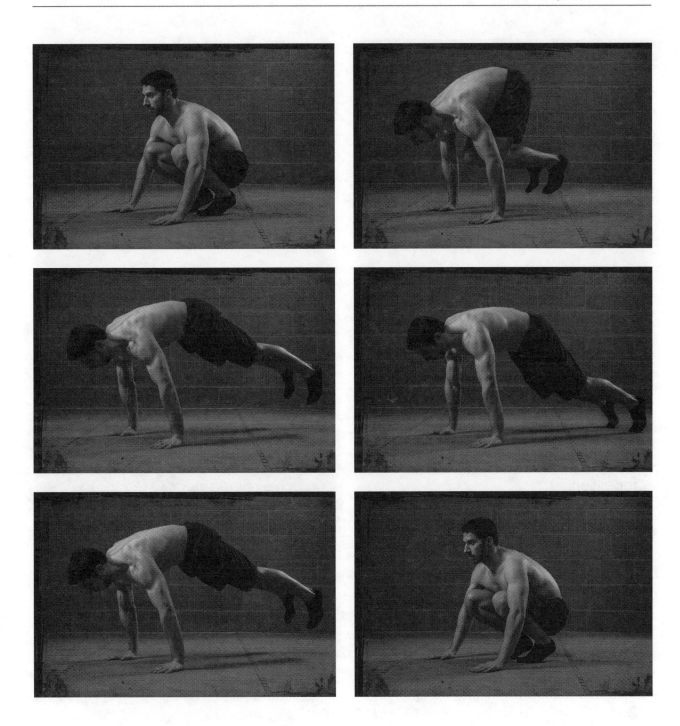

Mountain Climbers

Mountain climbers are yet another good conditioning exercise that can be used to increase fitness and burn body fat in a very effective way. They are very similar in principle to the squat thrust, and can simply be thought of as a one-legged variation of that exercise. They are also easier than the squat thrust so you should be able to do more of them.

1. Start in a push-up position but place one foot near to the hands. Keep the arms as straight as you can.

2. From here, jump into the air and switch legs, so that the front leg goes to the back and the back leg goes to the front.

3. From here, jump up and repeat the action so that your legs end up in the start position. This counts as one repetition.

Teaching Points

Try and perform 3 sets of 30 to 40 repetitions as fast as you can, and as many repetitions in a specific time period as possible. For example, see how many repetitions you can achieve in 3 sets of 60 seconds.

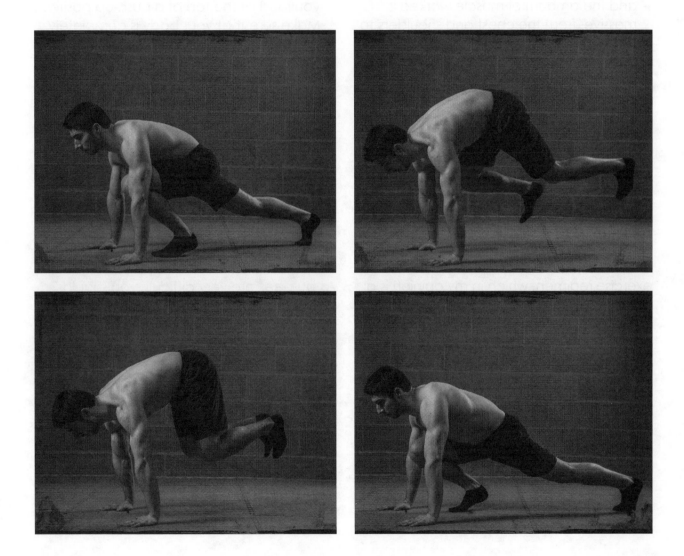

Burpees

Burpees are perhaps the most tiring of all conditioning exercises for three main reasons:

• The first is that the whole body is used, and the amount of muscle worked is massive, from the chest and shoulders to the core and legs.

• The second is that they should be performed as quickly as possible, which means that you will soon be gasping for breath.

• The third is that you have to move the body through space in two different ways, both backwards and forwards, and up and down.

Many people leave burpees out of their exercise regimen, which in my opinion is a massive mistake. They elicit such a huge response in the body that I frequently tell my clients that if they could only do one exercise to get fit, it would be the burpee.

1. Start in the crouched position, as you did with the squat thrust.

2. From here, jump your feet into the air and extend your legs out backwards until you land at the top of a push-up position. Make sure that your body is completely stretched out.

3. Next, jump your feet into the air and return them to the crouched position.

4. Finally, jump into the air as high as possible. As soon as you land, return to the crouched position. This counts as one repetition.

Teaching Points

As burpees are very difficult, you should start by attempting 3 sets of 10 repetitions. This should be plenty to begin your burpee training, and then increase the number as you become fitter and more conditioned.

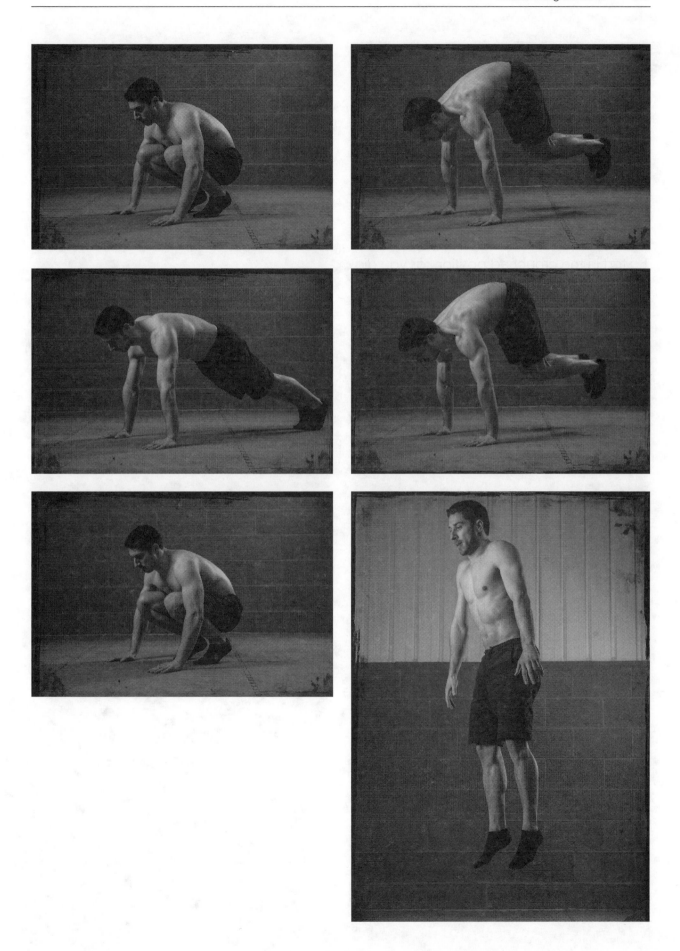

Bastards

Once you have familiarised yourself with the burpee, you can step it up a notch and perform a movement affectionately called the bastard. These are the same as the burpee in every way, except that when you arrive in the push-up position, you perform a push-up before returning your feet to the crouched position.

1. Start in the crouched position, as you did with the squat thrust.

2. From here, jump your feet into the air and extend your legs out backwards until you land at the top of a push-up position.

3. Once in the push-up position, perform a push-up.

4. After you have performed the push-up, jump your feet into the air and return them to the crouched position.

5. Now jump into the air as high as possible. As soon as you land, return to the crouched position. This counts as one repetition.

Teaching Points

Again, the bastard is a very challenging movement so you should start by only doing 3 sets of 8 to 10 repetitions. Increase this number as your fitness improves.

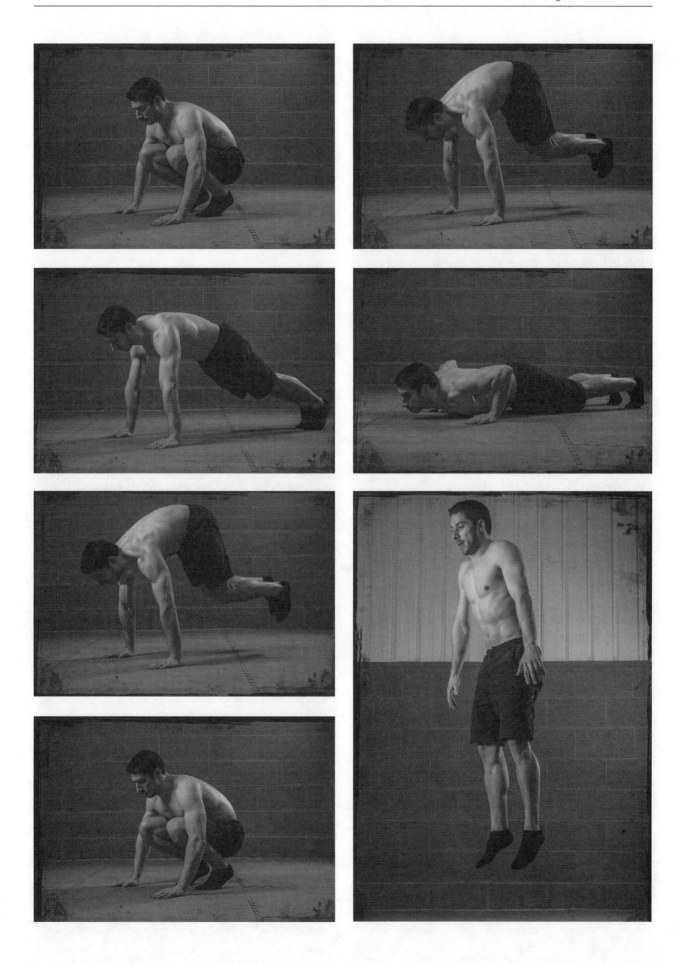

Sprints

Sprinting is perhaps one of the best whole body workouts you can possibly engage in, especially if you are looking for increased muscle mass, increased growth hormone output, and increased metabolism. There is a good reason why sprinters and marathon runners have such vastly different physiques, and it is not all down to diet. Sprinting and all other very high intensity exercise elicit huge changes in the body not only during the workout, but afterwards as well. It is this post-exercise energy expenditure that helps to shed body fat and encourages lean body mass maintenance.

There a few ways that you can perform sprints, but the two methods that I use are flat sprints and hill sprints. Flat sprints are performed on flat ground, such as a running track, grassland, or even a clear pavement or road. Hill sprints involve running up a hill as fast as possible. This is perhaps the most simple and tiring of all exercise activities, and will require not only strength of body but also strength of mind. In each case, make sure the area that you are running on is clear of debris and obstacles, and that there is no risk of you running into anybody.

1. To perform sprints simply increase your running pace to its maximum intensity. This means running as fast as your legs will go. You may have to build up to this but persevere.

2. Make sure to use your arms and put as much power into every movement as you can.

Teaching Points

In terms of sets and repetitions, try and sprint for a short period for a number of sets. For example, one of my best-loved distances to sprint is 40 to 50 meters. I will do this 5 times with at least 60 seconds rest after each sprint. Increase this distance to no more than 100 meters and try and keep the number of sets below 10, otherwise you will be too tired to sprint and the benefit will not be felt.

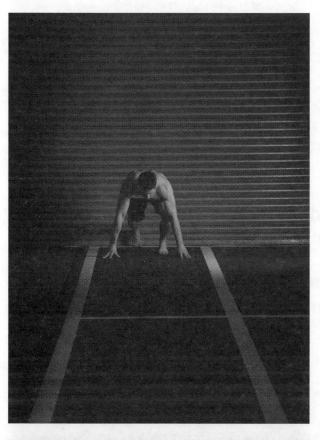

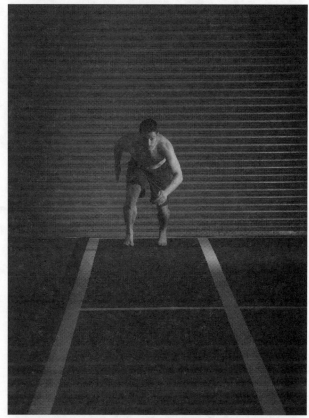

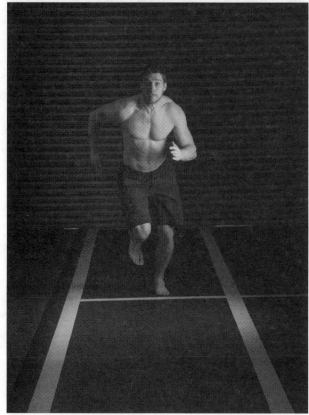

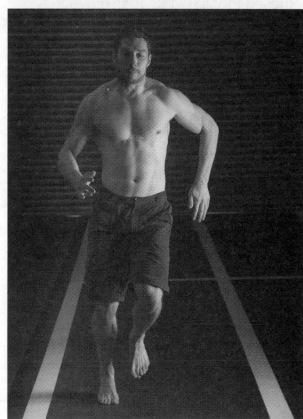

Bear Crawls

Bear crawls were considered a punishment exercise during the time that I spent training in the Royal Marines. Punishingly brutal, but utterly effective, bear crawls give the entire body a workout, involving all muscle groups, and really test your determination to the limit. Ideally you will need a patch of grass or other area where you can place your hands on the ground without fear of hurting or cutting them.

1. Get into a push-up position with your hands and feet slightly in front of one another. Make sure you keep your hips as low as you can, as you can see in the pictures.

2. From here, crawl forwards on your hands and feet, moving opposite hands and feet alternately. For example, as you move the right hand forwards, move the left foot forwards, then move the left hand forwards and the right foot forwards, etc. Continue like this for the desired distance or time. You can also crawl backwards for an added challenge.

Teaching Points

In terms of sets and repetitions, try and crawl for a set distance for 3 to 5 sets. For example, even 20 meters is a good distance to go, and you can also crawl for a set amount of time. For example, do 5 sets of 20 meters, or 5 sets of 40 seconds as far as you can.

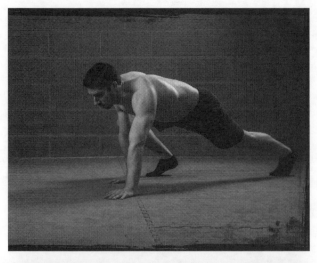

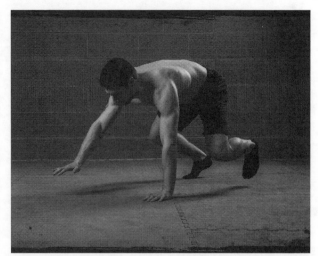

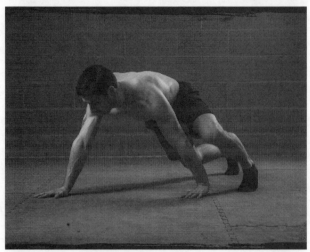

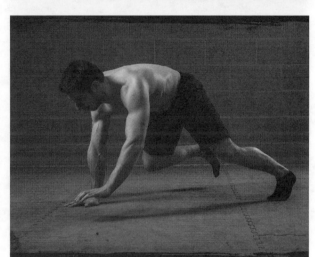

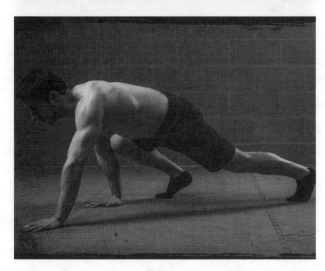

V Training Programs

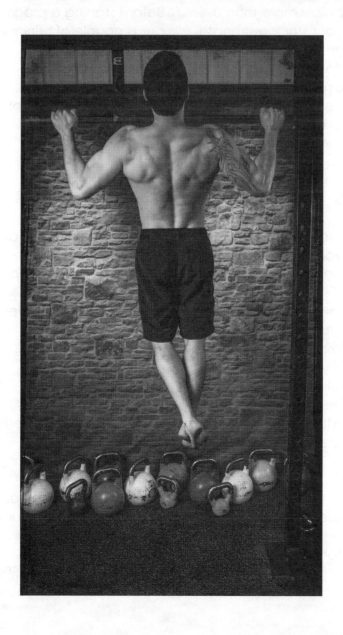

Now that we have looked at all of the available exercises, it is time to begin putting them into a program that we can follow and progress with. I will say at the outset that there is no such thing as a perfect program. Many people search for years in an attempt to find a program that will turn them from a weak, skinny individual into a strong, muscular one, but the simple fact is that such a program does not exist. All programs have the ability to work, and all that is preventing them from doing so is that people do not follow them for long enough. For example, learning and getting strong enough to perform a planche can take possibly more than a year, depending on your starting strength, training history, and genetics. If you only stick with a program for a few weeks, then you will never see the results, especially if the program has been designed to be followed for a number of months or more.

For a number of reasons, it is also impossible for me to produce programs that work well for everybody. Firstly, everybody has a unique genetic coding which determines many factors, including starting strength, mobility, how well your body deals with stress, how fast you recover, how your body adapts, etc. All that a program can offer is to give you guidance on how you should approach your training. Ultimately it is your responsibility to fine-tune your program to fit your own needs. Do not worry, I will explain fully how to do this, and also how to adapt and change it as you progress.

Before starting a program however, there are a couple of principles to bear in mind:

1. Establish your goal

2. Know the number of sets and repetitions for each exercise

Setting Goals

Establish your goal before you begin training; it may take you a little while to figure out, and it will undoubtedly change as you progress.

Although the overall theme of this book is to build as much strength and athletic potential as possible by using bodyweight exercises in a progressive manner, this does not mean that we cannot achieve other goals using calisthenics. A short list of possible goals might be as follows:

• Increased strength

• Increased muscle size

• Increased muscle tone and reduced body fat

• Increased mobility and flexibility

• Increased athletic potential

• Increased health benefits

• Stress reduction

• Social reasons

• Improving sports performance

• Rehabilitation and injury prevention

The goals listed are not exhaustive, but there will be at least one or two that apply to many of you.

Once you have identified your initial goal, I recommend that you write it down. This helps to solidify the goal and sets it in your mind and consciousness, and you are much more likely to follow it through. Next, write down the process by which you will achieve your goal. For physical training and calisthenics, the overarching factors are the amount of time you spend training, and the intensity at which you train. So for example, if your goal is to become stronger, then you could note that you intend to train for 5 days a week. If your goal is to perfect a handstand, then it should include at least 30 minutes of handstand practice every day. The important point to remember is that there is no definitive correct answer. This will vary and change according to the person and their exercise background, as well as many other factors that are outside of your control, including genetics, injuries, etc.

After you have written down your goal(s), it is time to make it into a SMART goal. The acronym SMART stands for; *Specific, Measurable, Achievable, Realistic,* and *Time-targeted.* As an example of goal-setting, let's say that my goal is to be able to perform 5 pull-ups within 3 months. Shown below is the way in which you would write this down.

- This is **Specific**, because it mentions the goal very clearly.

- It is **Measurable**, because I can simply test if I can perform 5 pull-ups.

- It is **Achievable**, because the methods to learning a pull-up are straightforward, and I can follow the progressions laid out in Part IV of this book.

- It is **Realistic**, because I will train 3 times a week, I will train hard, and I am determined to achieve the goal.

- It is **Time-targeted**, as I have allowed myself 3 months in which to reach my goal.

Shown next is an example of my goal-setting process. Bear in mind that this is *my* goal and is not necessarily the same as your goal.

- **Goal** – Increase strength, reduce body fat percentage, and progress onto more and more advanced calisthenic movements.

- **Process** – Train 4 to 5 times a week, depending on time and work commitments. Include equal amounts of pushing, pulling, core, and lower body exercises. Do more of one area if I feel I am getting weak or lacking in that part of the body.

- **Time-target** – Ongoing. Specific exercises will be tested at 6-monthly intervals.

Once you have this written down, then read the next section, which explains about sets, repetitions and hold times within the exercises themselves.many sets and repetitions to do and also how long to hold certain positions for. These numbers can be used to great effect, but it is important that you know why those particular numbers have been chosen.

Sets, Repetitions and Hold Times

In this part we will aim to understand more about sets, repetitions and hold times. You will have noticed that after each exercise in Part IV there is a short description of how many sets and repetitions to perform, and also for how long to hold certain positions. These numbers can be used to great effect, but it is important that you know why these particular numbers have been chosen.

For many years it has been well-understood that the number of repetitions, or the amount of time that your muscles are under tension, will dictate how your body reacts and adapts to the demands placed upon it. For example, for the body to become stronger, the resistance it works against needs to increase over time. There is little point in simply performing increasing numbers of repetitions, unless the overall resistance has increased. The same happens if you are trying to build muscular endurance but only work with low numbers of repetitions: your body will simply have no reason to increase its stamina.

Sets

The number of sets you perform will again depend on your goals. If you are looking to build strength, then you should perform only 2 to 4 sets per exercise, as the movements you will be performing could be very challenging and there will be a lot of stress and demand on the body. This means that you will not be able to keep performing sets for as long as you wish without getting fatigued.

If you are looking to build muscle size and mass, then I would recommend anything from 3 to 6 sets per exercise, as the movements you will be performing will be a little less stressful than for building strength.

For muscular endurance and increasing the number of repetitions that you can perform, you should try and do as many sets as is realistically possible, so anything from 5 to 10. Also, a technique called **Greasing the Groove** is very good at increasing the number of repetitions that you can perform of a given exercise. The way this works is to perform a *high* number of sets but a *low* number of repetitions within each set. For example, let's say that I wish to increase the number of pull-ups I can perform in one go. Try and complete something like 20 sets of 2 repetitions, so that you will be performing the pull-up movement many times, but will not become fatigued easily because you are only doing 2 repetitions within each set. Over time, you will become much more proficient at whatever exercise you choose, and your repetition range will increase dramatically.

Repetitions

How many repetitions you perform in each set is maybe the biggest dictator of how your body will adapt and react to the demands placed upon it. There are many different opinions on this subject, and you are just as likely to disagree with mine as anybody else's. However, there are some facts that are undeniable, which can be best represented by a few short lines:

• To build strength =
  Repetition range of 1 to 5

• To build muscle =
  Repetition range of 6 to 12

• To build muscular endurance =
  Repetition range of above 12

In essence, the less repetitions your body is able to perform of an exercise, the more strength it builds, and the more repetitions you can perform, the more muscular endurance it builds. This is not a hard and fast rule though, and it is often wise to experiment with different ranges and find out what works for you.

For many of the easier movements, it is possible to perform more repetitions quite easily, but once you find yourself doing some of the more challenging exercises, you will find that it is nearly impossible to perform many repetitions. For example, it is not uncommon to be able to perform upwards of 50 repetitions of normal push-ups, but I don't know of anybody who can perform the same number of planche push-ups. It is worth bearing this in mind when evaluating exactly how many repetitions you should be capable of in an exercise.

Hold Times

In contrast to sets and repetitions, hold times are somewhat different, as it is hard to quantify exactly how hard someone is contracting their muscles, although there are a few rules that we can follow. I have already mentioned that movements like the half lever should be performed for a specific time frame, say 30 seconds, in as many sets as it takes you. This is a good guide and enables your body to become accustomed to the exercise before you progress.

It goes without saying that some movements are so difficult that hold times of 30 seconds are simply not possible. For example, I think the world record for the planche is slightly longer than 20 seconds. However, this is not a bad thing. All it tells me is that the planche is a very difficult exercise and that because the hold time is so short, it is taking massive amounts of strength to perform. It is worth remembering this whenever you feel that your hold times are not long enough.

Over- and Undertraining

Among the many concerns for people starting a new form of exercise or exercise program, the main one has to be that either they will not train enough, so undertrain, or that they will train too much, so overtrain.

Undertraining is not necessarily a problem, as the only consequence is that you may not progress as quickly as you potentially could. Only you will know if you have more left in the tank to allow you to give a little more effort to an exercise. You should try and get to know your body to enable you to tell when you have done either enough or too much.

On the contrary, overtraining, if left unchecked, can ruin your progress and sideline you with various injuries and other problems. Remember, even though you are working with your own bodyweight, the stress and strain that your body will be under during some of the more challenging movements is very extreme and if you are not careful, you can injure yourself. This is much more likely to happen if you rush into movements for which you are not ready. Above all else, take your time and allow your body to become stronger. It will not happen overnight, but it *will* happen, so please be patient.

Creating Your Own Movements

The exercises and movements that I have shown and demonstrated so far are excellent in themselves, but your workouts can be taken to the next level by stringing and linking together different movements. There are unlimited ways of doing this, and the only real barrier is your imagination. Of course, with so many exercises available and so many potential combinations, it would be impossible for me to list all of them. This is reflected in the simplicity of the training programs that are shown towards the end of this section. What I can do though is to give you a few examples in the hope that it will spur your imagination and encourage you to experiment with your own training.

Example 1

The first example requires you to perform a close grip push-up, then a push-up, then a wide grip push-up, before starting again with the close grip push-up. Continue like this for the desired number of repetitions.

Example 2

In the second example, perform a dish for 10 seconds, then perform 5 v-ups, hold the dish again for 10 seconds, perform 5 v-ups, and so on, until you are fully exhausted.

Example 3

Perform 5 pull-ups and then perform 5 hanging leg raises. On the final leg raise move your legs through your arms and move into a back lever. Hold the back lever for as long as you can and then drop off the bar.

Example 4

Perform a single clap push-up, then a back clap push-up, then a double clap push-up, and finally a triple clap push-up. Repeat for as many repetitions as you can.

Example 5

Perform 3 single-leg squats, place the other foot down and jump as high and as far forwards as you can. Land, and then perform 3 single-leg squats with the opposite leg. Repeat for 3 to 5 sets.

Example 6

Hang from a bar and perform a single pull-up. At the top of the movement move into a front lever, then move back to the top portion of a pull-up again. Then lower down to a dead hang again. Repeat for as many repetitions as you can.

Example 7

Get into an extended plank and move your hands as far away from your feet as possible. Hold the extended plank for 10 seconds, and then allow your body to drop to the ground. Perform 5 Lalanne push-ups, and then shuffle your hands back towards your feet until you are in a push-up position. Repeat for as many sets as you can.

Example 8

Hang from a bar with an overhand grip. Perform a hanging leg raise. Now perform a German hang and hold the position for 10 seconds. Then move your legs through the gap in your arms into a dead hang again. Repeat for 3 sets of as many repetitions as possible.

Example 9

Perform a false grip muscle-up and pause at the top of the movement. Now perform 5 front dips. Now do a very slow negative muscle-up, and then drop off when your reach the dead hang position. These count as one set.

Example 10

Get into a freestanding handstand and hold for 5 seconds. Perform as many handstand push-ups as possible and then walk as far as you can on your hands.

The examples I have just given are the tip of the iceberg. Depending on your strength level, the equipment that is available, or your training goals, there are literally millions of combinations of exercises that you can perform when you use a little imagination. On top of all of that, you can even create your own exercises. Free your mind, and don't feel any constraints on your physical ability!

Now that we have the background information you need for goal-setting, sets, repetitions and hold times, it is time to start looking at the training programs themselves. There are four different *Complete Calisthenics* programs that are designed to take you from beginner, and beyond.

Program 1 Fundamental Five

The first program we are going to look at is called the Fundamental Five. This program is designed to make sure that the foundation exercises that I listed on page 76, the push-up, pull-up, triceps dip, hanging knee raise, and squat, can be performed perfectly with no technical errors. As I explained before, this is a vital stage, and I would recommend ensuring that you can perform all of these movements perfectly before moving on to the more advanced exercises.

This is a beginner-level program. Some of you that have either trained before or who consider yourself as having a decent level of strength should still try to meet these requirements before moving onto the next program. The requirements are:

• **Push-ups – 20 perfect repetitions**

• **Pull-ups – 10 perfect repetitions**

• **Triceps dips – 10 perfect repetitions**

• **Hanging knee raises – 10 perfect repetitions**

• **Squats – 25 perfect repetitions**

You might think that only working up to five exercises might be somewhat boring, and in reality it can be, but this stage is essential if you have only just started training or you cannot perform the movements as demonstrated. If you do not lay the proper foundations you will always struggle to progress. For most people, even complete beginners, it should not take too long to be able to complete all of the exercises in this section, so stay determined and keep pushing forwards. There are easier exercises than the five I have listed here, such as the box dip, row, chin-up, plank, dish, crunch, side plank, lunge, calf raise, etc., and you should include these in your training as well. It is important to remember however, that the main purpose is to increase strength so that the higher-level exercises can be reached, and this means that if an exercise is too easy for you, simply move on.

In terms of which muscles to work on which days, it is not really necessary to divide your training into specific body parts, like a bodybuilder. We are training movement patterns, and as the exercises are roughly divided into pushing, pulling, core, lower body, and conditioning, it makes sense to keep them that way for our training program as well. As a beginner we do not want to overtrain either, so a maximum of four training days per week will be more than sufficient.

The following table outlines the *Fundamental Five* program that you can use as a guide to help plan your workout. It is divided into a 7-day rotating workout that starts on Monday with pushing exercises for the upper body. This routine should be followed by even the most inexperienced person, and will deliver good gains in strength and proficiency if it is followed properly and the exercise techniques performed correctly.

Again, it is recommended that you perform a good mobility workout before your actual strength workout, and make sure to stretch afterwards (see Chapter 4).

Day	Exercise / Sets / Repetitions / Other Information
Monday	**Push-ups** – 3 sets of as many repetitions as you can manage **Ledge dips/triceps dips** – 3 sets of as many repetitions as you can manage **Squats/lunges** – 3 sets of as many repetitions as you can manage **Conditioning exercises** – (if you want to do them)
Tuesday	**Rows/chin-ups** – 3 sets of as many repetitions as you can manage **Plank/lying leg ext./hanging knee raise/etc.** – 3 sets of as many repetitions as you can manage
Wednesday	Rest day
Thursday	**Push-ups** – 3 sets of as many repetitions as you can manage **Ledge dips/triceps dips** – 3 sets of as many repetitions as you can manage **Squats/lunges** – 3 sets of as many repetitions as you can manage **Conditioning exercises** – (if you want to do them)
Friday	**Rows/chin-ups** – 3 sets of as many repetitions as you can manage **Plank/lying leg ext./hanging knee raise/etc.** – 3 sets of as many repetitions as you can manage
Saturday	Rest day
Sunday	Rest day

Monday

The first exercise is the push-up. Try and perform 3 sets and as many repetitions as you can in each set. It is fine if you use a raised platform for the hands as we are just trying to increase strength for now.

The second exercise is the dip exercise. Here you can do either a ledge dip if you have insufficient strength, or some triceps dips if your strength is at a decent level. Keep trying to work towards the goal of doing 10 perfect triceps dips.

Thirdly you will perform 3 sets of squats. Concentrate on good form and try and descend as low as possible. Your target is to be able to perform 25 perfect repetitions before moving on.

You can also do conditioning exercises as well if that is part of your goal, although this is not essential, as our main focus for now is to build strength.

Tuesday

Your aim now is to perform a pulling exercise, ideally the chin-up. If you are not strong enough to perform any chin-ups, work with the row until your strength increases. Again, you should be aiming for 3 sets of as many repetitions as you can, until you can do 10 perfect repetitions.

The second exercise should be your core exercise. This can be any of the easier variations, such as the plank, crunch, dish, or hanging leg raise. Remember that the sole aim here is to work up to performing 10 perfect hanging knee raises.

Wednesday

This is a rest day, so ensure that you get plenty of good food and sleep.

Thursday

This should be the same as Monday's workout.

Friday

This should be the same as Tuesday's workout.

Saturday/Sunday

These are both rest days, as in the beginning it is important for your body to have enough rest and to be able to recover properly from the workouts. This also leaves you completely fresh for the week ahead.

As was said before, only once you can perform the five fundamental movements and their required number of repetitions, should you move on to the next program.

Program 2 Building on the Basics

After you have mastered the movements listed in the *Fundamental Five* program, move onto some of the more challenging variations shown in the exercise section. The second program is called *Building on the Basics*, because in effect this is exactly what you will be doing.

For this program we will be looking at incorporating some of the more advanced variations of each exercise type. For example, wide grip push-ups, wide grip pull-ups, front dips, hanging leg raises, etc.

Another exercise group used in this program are the handstands. It does not matter if this is only the first or second stage of the handstand, like wall walks or a wall-supported handstand, just so long as your shoulders and upper body become exposed to the stresses and strains that this type of exercise places upon them.

The overall goal of this program is to keep building strength and to prepare your body for the much more difficult movements. With that in mind, there are no real requirements other than to become accustomed to performing plenty of different variations of the exercises. This does not mean that you have to do all of the movements and learn every single exercise before moving on; it simply means that you need to expose the body to enough stress that it changes and becomes stronger.

Feel free to insert any conditioning movements you may wish to include on any day where you can fit them in.

Day	Exercise / Sets / Repetitions / Other Information
Monday	**Push-up variations** – Wide grip push-ups, clap push-ups, etc. Go for 3 or 4 sets of each and try and do as many repetitions as you can. Make sure to stick to the correct number of sets and repetitions for your goals. For example, if you are training for pure strength then go for a low numbers of repetitions and only 3 to 4 sets **Dip variations** – Triceps dips, front dips, etc. Again, go for numbers that will help you to build as much strength as possible. There is no real requirement here, just keep progressing and get stronger **Core variations** – Hanging leg raises, side plank, v-ups, dragon flags, etc. Try and include as many different types of core exercises as possible, and go for maximum strength rather than lots of repetitions. Remember, tension in the muscles here is key
Tuesday	**Pull-up/muscle-up variations** – Wide grip pull-ups, rock climbers, muscle-ups, etc. Concentrate on good form and try and engage the correct muscles **Lower body exercise variations** – Lunges, deep squats, single-leg squats, etc. Just try and get some repetitions done here. Good range of motion on the exercises will give the most benefit **Handstand work** – Start work with wall walks and then on kicking up into a handstand against a wall. You can use the floor and parallels here if you have them. Spend at least 20 minutes practicing this
Wednesday	Rest day
Thursday	This is the same as Monday's training day
Friday	This is the same as Monday's training day
Saturday	Rest day
Sunday	Rest day

You can see from the table, that as with the previous program, the workout is split into a 7-day routine.

Monday

On the first training day you should perform push-up variations, dip variations, and core variations. Exactly which exercises you perform is your choice, but as a short guide, I would recommend the following; close grip, wide grip, and deep push-ups, triceps dips, front dips, hanging leg raises, side planks, v-ups, and dragon flags. We are trying to build as much strength as possible at this stage, so keep with low numbers of sets and a low to moderate number of repetitions for each exercise.

Tuesday

This is the next training day where you will be performing pull-up and muscle-up variations, lower body movements, as well as starting some handstand work for the first time.

For the pull-up variations, try chin-ups, pull-ups, and wide grip pull-ups to begin with, before moving onto more demanding variations. Remember, it is all about building as much strength as possible so keep the muscles under tension and keep your form as good as you can. For the muscle-ups you should simply be trying to make your pull to the bar stronger, as well as working a little bit on the transition stage of the movement. Do not worry if it feels as if you are not making much progress; this takes time, so be patient – it will happen.

For the lower body movements it is advisable to start working on lunges, deep squats, and the bridge, etc. Your legs should be naturally stronger and you should not struggle too much with the lower body movements until you get to the single-leg squat and the hamstring curl. This day should also include some handstand work, and for most people, this will consist of wall walks and possibly wall-supported handstands. Make sure that you spend some time practicing your handstands as they build huge levels of strength and athletic ability with a little investment of time and effort.

Wednesday

This is a rest day where you should try and eat as much good quality food as possible and also have plenty of good quality sleep.

Thursday

This is a repeat of Monday, where push-up variations, dip variations, and pull-up variations are performed.

Friday

This day is a repeat of Tuesday, where core exercise variations, lower body exercise variations, and handstand work should be completed.

Saturday/Sunday

These are both rest days, where you should try and eat as much good quality food as possible and also have plenty of good quality sleep.

As there are no requirements for this program, I would simply suggest that you become comfortable performing some of the average-level exercises with ease before moving onto the next program, *Learning the Levers*. This is because the levers are much more difficult than the *Fundamental Five*, and therefore you will need to build a good base of strength before progressing.

Program 3 Learning the Levers

Once you have become proficient with some of the more advanced movements, then you can begin to incorporate the static holds and levers into your training. This third program is known as *Learning the Levers*. Here you will be exposed to the planche, front lever, back lever, half lever, and the human flag. All of these are isometric exercises, which are extremely taxing on the body, not only in a muscular sense, but also in the way that they stress the nervous system. Holding the body in a locked position where all of the muscle groups are contracting hard can really take its toll, in much the same way as performing heavy bench presses, deadlifts, and weighted squats, and the first few workouts may come as a shock.

In this program, you will not simply be performing the levers and nothing else (although that program would yield incredible gains), but you will be adding them to your normal training. This means that you will still do push-up variations, pull-ups variations, dips, muscle-ups, core exercises, squats, etc., as well as starting to work with all five of the levers. You will also be practicing 5 to 10 minutes of handstands at almost every session. This is because, as well as being a strength exercise, handstands require huge amounts of skill, and to develop this, you simply need to practice them.

I do not really see the need to include some of the easier core exercises, because most of the levers make use of the core very intensely, and performing the easier core movements will yield little to no benefit strength-wise.

Again, feel free to insert any conditioning movements you may wish to include on any day where you can fit them in.

Day	Exercise / Sets / Repetitions / Other Information
Monday	**Planche work** – Start right at the beginning and only move on when you are ready. Strive to achieve perfect form at each stage **Pull-up variations** – Strive to perform the hardest variations that you can **Handstands** – 5 to 10 minutes practice
Tuesday	**Back lever work** – Start right at the beginning and only move on when you are ready. Strive to achieve perfect form at each stage **Dip variations** – Strive to perform the hardest variations that you can **Handstands** – 5 to 10 minutes practice
Wednesday	Rest day
Thursday	**Front lever work** – Start right at the beginning and only move on when you are ready. Strive to achieve perfect form at each stage **Push-up variations** – Strive to perform the hardest variations that you can **Handstands** – 5 to 10 minutes practice
Friday	**Human flag work** – Start right at the beginning and only move on when you are ready. Strive to achieve perfect form at each stage **Muscle-ups** – Make sure to include the false grip variation here and work especially hard on the transition **Handstands** – 5 to 10 minutes practice Half lever work – Start right at the beginning and only move on when you are ready. Strive to achieve perfect form at each stage
Saturday	**Half lever work** – Start right at the beginning and only move on when you are ready. Strive to achieve perfect form at each stage **Lower body exercises** – By this stage you should be working towards some of the more difficult lower body exercises, such as the single-leg squat, deep squat, and hamstring curl
Sunday	Rest day

As with programs 1 and 2, program 3 is broken down into 7-day blocks.

Monday

On the first training day you will begin with planche work. If you are completely new to calisthenics, then planche leans and frog stands are 'where it's at', as these will expose you to the demands of planche training whilst building strength in a progressive manner. In contrast to the planche, you will also perform pull-ups, so that you incorporate both pushing and pulling into a single training session. You should strive to perform the most difficult pull-up variations that you can, and try and perform a couple of different types. You will also spend some time doing handstands.

Tuesday

On the second training day you will begin by looking at the back lever. It is important that you start with the German hang stage, as this will get your shoulders accustomed to being in the unusual position required by the back lever. As the back lever is a pulling-based exercise, you will do dips on this day as well, so that you balance the push with the pull. Again, as with Monday, you will also do some handstand work to ensure that you keep progressing with the skill.

Wednesday

The third day in this program is a rest day.

Thursday

On the fourth day you will be doing front lever work; if you have some pull-up strength, then the first stage of these should not be problematic, but the movement is still very challenging. You will also perform push-up variations, and these should be the most difficult ones that you can currently manage. Again, at some point in the session, you should perform some handstand work to keep building your skill and proficiency.

Friday

The fifth day in this program includes training for the human flag. This is another very difficult movement, and as such you should begin with the easiest variation and progress as you become stronger. You will also include muscle-up work, which will help to reinforce shoulder and scapula strength. Again, at some point in the session, you should perform some handstand work to keep building your skill and proficiency.

Saturday

The last training day in the program should include the half lever as the main exercise. Start with the tuck variation, aiming to progressively work towards the raised or full version. On this day you will also include lower body movements, working towards the single-leg squat and the hamstring curl. Again, at some point in the session, you should perform some handstand work to keep building your skill and proficiency.

Sunday

The last day in the program is a rest day.

Program 4 Complete Calisthenics

Once you have progressed with the levers and have begun to graduate towards some of the more advanced movements in the other chapters, it will be time to move onto the last program, which I have named *Complete Calisthenics*. By the time you reach this program, you should have a very high level of strength, and it is now that you can finally progress onto the most difficult exercises in the book. In this program more than any other, it is vital and recommended that you try as often as possible to string movements together to create combinations and exercises of your own.

Note that the program I have produced here can, and only ever will be, a guide. I have chosen to include the greatest spread of exercises possible, but if you choose to concentrate on one specific area, e.g. the planche or the one-arm pull-up, then this is absolutely fine.

The *Complete Calisthenics* program is about striving towards the high-level movements and exercises within this book. By this point you should have a very good idea of the number of sets, repetitions and hold times per exercise, and this is why there are not any included in this section. In addition, by the time you have progressed to this program, you will have your own ideas about exactly what you wish to accomplish. Do not feel obliged to perform some of the movements I have written down, as you may have one particular area of your physique or strength you wish to work on, e.g. your back or your pushing strength.

Again, feel free to insert any conditioning movements you may wish to include on any day where you can fit them in.

Day	Exercise / Sets / Repetitions / Other Information
Day 1	**Pushing movements** – Planche, handstand work, and very high-level push-up variations. Try and combine the movements together into different circuits. You should be aiming continuously to be working towards the most advanced exercises. The sets, repetitions, and hold times that you perform here should be aligned with your own specific goals
Day 2	**Pulling movements** – Front levers, back levers, and the high level pull-up variations. Try and combine the movements together into different circuits. You should be aiming continuously to be working towards the most advanced exercises. The sets, repetitions, and hold times that you perform here should be aligned with your own specific goals
Day 3	Rest day
Day 4	**Core exercises** – Half lever, dragon flag, hanging leg raises, etc. Try and combine the movements together into different circuits. You should be aiming continuously to be working towards the most advanced exercises. The sets, repetitions, and hold times that you perform here should be aligned with your own specific goals
Day 5	**Lower body and conditioning exercises** – Single-leg squat variations, hamstring curls, burpees, jump squats, etc. Try and combine the movements together into different circuits. You should be aiming continuously to be working towards the most advanced exercises. The sets, repetitions, and hold times that you perform here should be aligned with your own specific goals
Day 6	Rest day

For this program, the routine is split into a 6-day cycle that simply rotates around before returning to the beginning. For example, if you began this program at the beginning of the week, Monday would be day 1 through to Saturday, which would be day 6. Then Sunday would be day 1 again, Monday would be day 2, and so on. Obviously, it may not be possible to actually keep to this schedule for many different reasons, so if you cannot avoid taking two rest days, then simply pick up the program where you left off.

You will notice in this program that you will only be doing one type of movement once every 6 days. Initially this may seem like a stupid idea, but as the high-level exercises generate so much muscular tension in the body, you will not need to do pushing movements every day, for example, to keep progressing.

Day 1

Day 1 is where you will perform all of the pushing movements in your program. Pushing movements are those that use the muscles that push; the chest, triceps, shoulders, forearms, and core. These exercises include planches, handstands, push-ups, and dips.

Day 2

Day 2 is where you will perform all of the pulling movements in your program. Pulling movements are those that use the muscles that pull; the back, shoulders, biceps, and forearms. These exercises include front levers, back levers, muscle-ups, and all of the advanced pull-up variations.

Day 3

Day 3 is your first designated rest day.

Day 4

Day 4 is where you will perform all of the core exercises in your program. As I have already mentioned, it is true that many of the pulling and pushing type exercises involve the core to a large degree, but there is nothing wrong with having a separate training day where you perform specific core strengthening exercises. You should concentrate on the following core exercises: the half lever, human flag, dragon flag, and any of the other high-level core movements.

Day 5

Day 5 is where you will perform all of your lower body strength work and also the conditioning exercises. The lower body includes all of the muscles that are used to run, jump, change direction, and most of the so-called athletic movements. The exercises in this section will be the high-level lower body exercises, e.g. the single-leg squat, hamstring curl, and high box jump. The high-level conditioning exercises include the burpee, the jump squat, and sprints.

Day 6

Day 6 is your second designated rest day. After this, you will start again at day 1.

Creating Your Own Program

As we are all individuals, it may be that the programs that I have set out in the previous sections are not completely applicable to you, or you may have strengths and weaknesses different to mine. To this end, it is important that you are able to learn how to create your own program so that you can perform the exercises that will be the most appropriate for your overall athletic development. For example, your pulling strength may be out of sync with your pushing strength, meaning that you will need to spend more time on the pulling movements to address this imbalance.

The programs that I have outlined are a very good place to start when it comes to designing your own, but before you do, you must ask yourself what it is that you are looking to accomplish. Have you got a specific exercise that you would like to perfect? Have you got a particular sport that you would like to increase your strength for? Are you geographically close to a gym? If not, have you the resources to buy equipment? Once you have answered those questions, it will be time to begin constructing your program.

- Initially, you should identify the amount of time you have to train. It is no good wanting to learn a one-arm chin-up in three months if you only have an hour a week in which to do so. For most people, even with full-time jobs and/or family commitments, a few hours a week should be sufficient time in which to start progressing.

- Secondly, you need to establish exactly what your goal is for the program. For example, a goal of mine a couple of years ago was to get my planche to a comfortable level. This meant that most of my training for a few months was geared around developing the strength to perform the planche.

- Thirdly, you should try and work out your current level of strength or fitness. This will involve simply working out which of the exercises you can perform. Once you have done this, then you can start to put movements into your program. For example, for my planche training program, I included push-ups to warm up with, flat back planches to get my nervous system firing properly, and then finally working with straddle planches and full planches until I achieved a total hold time of 60 seconds.

After this, you should have something resembling a program that you can follow as long as you need to. Once you have reached that specific goal, you can develop a new program to enable you to accomplish something new. Keep doing this as long as necessary.

Final Word

My sole aim of writing this book was to share my enthusiasm for bodyweight and calisthenic training with as many people as possible. I have experienced many different forms of training and exercise, and by far the most fun has been the journey that I have adventured on with calisthenics. Hopefully I have reassured and convinced you that an awesome physique, strength, and athleticism do not require magic pills or the newest piece of mega-expensive equipment. Your own bodyweight, consistent hard work, and patience are the only elements required.

In closing I would like to thank you, the reader, for buying this book and for helping to spread the message of calisthenic training throughout the world. In these days of corporations and huge multinational companies, it is all too easy to get sucked into the media's idea of what a strong and agile human being should look like, and all too often this is not the image that many of us desire. I would also encourage you not to rush through the book but to take your time with the movements. Becoming stronger, especially using calisthenics, takes time and dedication.

Frequently Asked Questions

Often, many people have questions that are not answered in the main portion of the book, so in this final section, we will look at some of the most commonly asked.

Q. Ashley, I am training hard, eating right, getting enough rest, etc., but do not seem to be progressing very quickly at all. What is going on?

A. Progression using these types of bodyweight movements has traditionally been seen as being easy, or quick, but the reality is that building enough strength to perform some of the more advanced movements is a long and arduous process.

Let us take the planche for example. This movement took me a good two years to achieve, and when I started I had a good level of strength. The same would be true of someone wanting to lift say 250kg or 500lbs in the deadlift. There is no way that this level of strength can be built in a short period of time. The muscles would need time to grow, the nervous system would need time to become stronger, and the tendons and ligaments would need time to adapt to the stress and demands placed upon them.

Any high-level movement can and will take months, if not years to develop the strength and ability to perform.

Q. Ashley, many people have told me that strength cannot be built with bodyweight exercise alone. Is this true?

A. This is absolutely not true, and for proof, simply look at a gymnast! They very rarely do any movements with weights, and they are perhaps the strongest athletes, pound for pound, on earth. The days are over where people do bodyweight exercise as

a warm-up, or simply do lots of repetitions. Not only can calisthenic and bodyweight exercise build high levels of strength, the strength that can be built is often much more useful than that built simply by doing body building movements.

Q. Ashley, some people have told me that some of the movements in this book, like handstands, are dangerous. Is this true?

A. Whilst some movements, like handstands and clapping pull-ups can be dangerous, it is very unlikely that you will become injured whilst performing them. The reason is that the more difficult exercises take time to build up to, and so simply cannot be attempted if you have a low level of strength.

For example, let us take a bench press. Any novice can jump on a bench and put 400lbs on the bar. If they are unprepared, then they may seriously injure themselves. This is true of all weighted exercises as it is possible for anyone, regardless of their level of experience or ability, to load up a bar or a machine with far too much weight for them to realistically handle.

Q. Ashley, are you against weight training altogether? I have seen plenty of benefits from training with weights, so why should I give up that method and style of training?

A. I am not saying that weightlifting is bad, only that bodyweight exercise can help to build a much better all-round physical structure and physique. This is why many of the top athletes in the world, even those whose primary goal is to lift weight, train using bodyweight exercises and calisthenics. The example I gave in the beginning was that of Lu Xiaojun and the other Olympic weightlifters.

In addition, many people simply lift weights to look better or to get bigger muscles. In my opinion, this is a very narrow training viewpoint. There is nothing wrong with wanting to look good, but surely one of the most rewarding outcomes of training is an increased physical capability and the ability to do things that other people cannot. As Mark Rippetoe has so eloquently explained in his book *Starting Strength*, strong people are more useful than weak people, and are much harder to kill.

Q. Ashley, I have had injuries and joint problems from training in the past. Will the movements in *Complete Calisthenics* aggravate them?

A. Many people have many different types of injury, and these can prevent some of those people from training or engaging in physical activities.

Calisthenics is unique in that the only weight you use as the resistance is that of your own bodyweight. This makes it inherently much safer than weighted exercise, as I have already explained. Not only that, but the manipulation of the leverage that is involved with some movements, like the levers, builds huge tendon and ligament strength, that you will struggle to build in other exercise regimens.

The likelihood is that you end up stronger, more agile, and much less injury-prone after starting calisthenics than you ever have in the past.

Q. Ashley, there is no periodisation in this book. Why is that?

A. Periodisation refers to the scaling of intensity within an exercise or training program. This is well-understood, and is carried out so that athletes can carry on progressing and not plateau or injure themselves. The problem with me stating exactly when you should reduce your training intensity, and for how long, is that I have no idea what your strength level or exercise history is. I also have no idea about the type and quality of food that you eat, and the amount and quality of your rest. As a very inaccurate guide, I would recommend that you experiment with a deloading, or lower training intensity week every 8 to 12 weeks or so. This is where you should simply reduce the amount and the intensity of your training to allow the body to recover fully.

The main point is to listen to your body, as it alone can tell you how often to rest, for how long, when to train more intensively, and when to have an easy workout. The longer you train, the better you will become at knowing when you need to do this.

Q. Ashley, I am really tempted to try some of the more advanced exercises, but I cannot perform the Fundamental Five that are required. What should I do?

A. Whatever you do, do not move on to the more advanced movements until you can perform the 5 exercises properly and for the correct number of repetitions. They are there for a reason, and need to be perfected so that you will have a solid base on which to build your strength. As I have said before, you should not run before you can walk, and the same applies here. It may be very tempting to progress faster than I have advised, but I have seen many people make the same mistake and they always regret it. Spend your time getting the basics right, and the rest will follow.

Q. I am not really that keen on training the lower body, and it seems like the legs are not needed for most of the more advanced exercises (planche, front lever, handstands, etc.). Can I simply leave the lower body out of my training routine?

A. You can, of course, remove leg exercises from your training, but I wouldn't recommend this for a number of reasons. Firstly, training the lower body can help to increase strength in the rest of the body as hormones are released that help the growth of muscle and strength when you train large muscle groups, like those in the lower body. Secondly, if you are interested in developing a complete physique, then it makes no sense to leave out one of the most important areas of the body. Training the legs makes it possible for you to run faster, jump higher, change direction more quickly, and just become more athletic in general.

Q. Ashley, I am very tall. Will the fact that my limbs are long make it more difficult for me to build strength using calisthenic and bodyweight exercise?

A. There is no doubt that if you have long arms and legs, then the force that you have to apply to perform some of the movements featured in this book will be more difficult. This is simply a matter of biomechanics. Long levers will always need to exert more force to achieve the same goal. For example, a tall person may take longer to achieve the full front lever than a shorter person. However, as a tall person, because you need to exert more force, ultimately you will be able to build more strength than a shorter person.

Above all else, do not try and come up with excuses to either not train, or to explain away your lack of progress. Remember, you are not in competition with anyone but yourself, and the only measure of success is how good you feel after achieving a goal that you have set for yourself.

Q. Ashley, I feel a bit stupid attempting calisthenic movements in my gym, as almost no one else does anything like this where I train. Do you have any suggestions?

A. There is always a time when you think that the training method you are using is a little bit strange, but remember, calisthenics is about trying to push the boundaries of what your body is capable of. If the guys standing in the weights area want to laugh at you from the safety of the dumbbell rack, let them. They will still be curling the 20s when you are smashing out repetitions of full range of motion handstand push-ups, and when you do, they will be coming to you for advice.

Q. Ashley, I do not really have an interest in the conditioning exercises. Do I have to perform them or can I leave them out and just concentrate on strength work?

A. As I have already explained in one of my previous answers, it is not a requirement that you include all of the movements I have presented in this book. If your goal is simply to develop as much strength as humanly possible, then it is completely fine to leave the conditioning exercises out of your routine. The conditioning movements are there to help to increase your fitness and resilience to fatigue, and can also help to burn body fat and make you look more ripped.

The conditioning exercises will also help to build mental strength. Movements such as burpees, jump squats, sprints, etc. are very taxing, not only on the physical system, but also on the mental and nervous systems. You will experience fatigue and tiredness and it is your mind that dictates whether you stop or not. Do not make the mistake of thinking that training is purely physical. The changes that occur to your body happen both inside and out, and sometimes it is the changes that happen on the inside that make the biggest difference to your life.

Q. Ashley, I am a female but I still want to train using calisthenics. Can women do this type of training?

A. Yes of course! One of the most apt quotes is from the health and wellbeing practitioner Paul Chek, who remarked that women are "equal, but not the same." What he meant is that whilst women in the modern world have become more and more equal in terms of influence, pay, social standing, etc., they are not the equivalent in terms of physical make-up. Women often have a much stronger lower body compared to their upper body, whereas in men it is often the other way around. Women are also not as naturally as strong as men. Fact.

This does not mean that as a woman you cannot perform the exercises in this book or be a great calisthenic practitioner, it just means that it may take you a little longer to reach your goal(s), so keep training!

In my own life, I have met and am friends with some incredibly strong women. Not only have they all built strength using bodyweight exercise, but some have excelled to levels that their male friends would not have thought possible.

Q. Ashley, I am also a woman that wants to get strong, but many of my female friends have said that doing any strength work will make my muscles get big. Is this true?

A. Whilst it is somewhat true that muscle does grow as a result of strength training, bodyweight exercise is not known for making people huge. In addition, women have far less testosterone (the male sex hormone) going around their bodies, so it is far more difficult for them to build muscle in the first place. Also, building lots of muscle (like female bodybuilders do) requires enormous amounts of food, specific training designed to make the muscles huge, and sometimes a little chemical help in the form of testosterone injections, growth hormone, and other anabolic steroids. To reiterate the question I have just answered, look at any female gymnast. They will be far stronger than the majority of men that you will meet in your everyday life and they are far from bulky or too muscular.

Major Skeletal Muscles

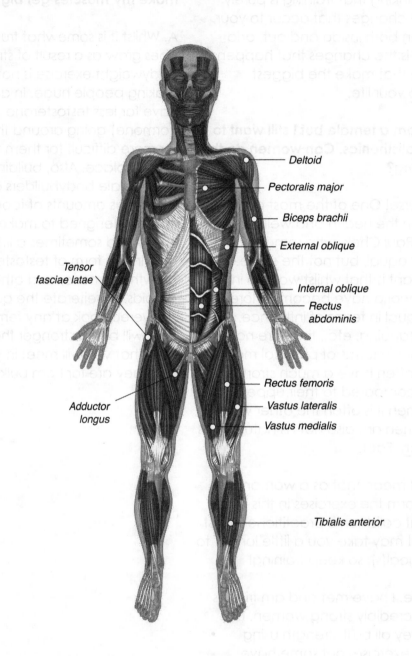

Deltoid

Pectoralis major

Biceps brachii

External oblique

Tensor
fasciae latae

Internal oblique

Rectus
abdominis

Rectus femoris

Adductor
longus

Vastus lateralis

Vastus medialis

Tibialis anterior

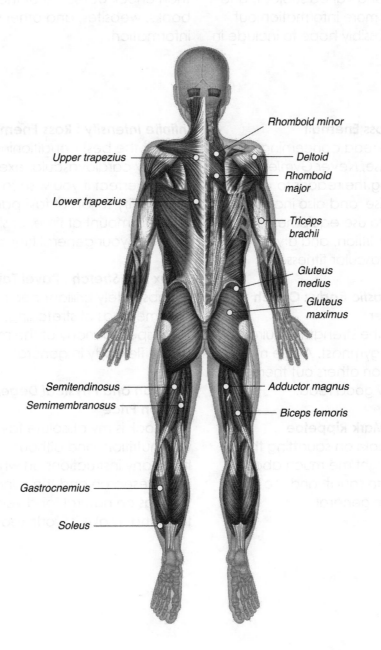

Rhomboid minor

Upper trapezius

Deltoid

Rhomboid major

Lower trapezius

Triceps brachii

Gluteus medius

Gluteus maximus

Semitendinosus

Adductor magnus

Semimembranosus

Biceps femoris

Gastrocnemius

Soleus

Resources

Calisthenics and strength training in general is a huge and varied subject, and as such there is far more information out there than I can possibly hope to include in this volume. If you would like to know more, then check out some of the following books, websites, and other sources of information.

Books

Never Gymless : **Ross Enemait**
The first book that I read concerning bodyweight exercise, *Never Gymless* is good for exposing the reader to bodyweight exercise, and also includes lots of novel ways to use equipment, a good section on nutrition, and a very good section on cardiovascular fitness.

Building the Gymnastic Body : **Coach Christopher Sommer**
Excellent book on the strength required by the beginner level gymnast. A little more textbook in style than others out there, but nevertheless a very good read.

Starting Strength : **Mark Rippetoe**
One of the best books on squatting that exists, this book taught me much about why it is important to squat, and the value of weight training in general.

Infinite Intensity : **Ross Enemait**
One of the best conditioning and high intensity cardiovascular exercise books out there, perfect if you wish to really increase your ability to lots of fast paced work in a short amount of time, or simply want to increase your general fitness.

Relax into Stretch : **Pavel Tatsouline**
An absolutely brilliant book on the science and methods of stretching, and for me this dispelled many of the myths that exist about flexibility in general.

Nutrition and Physical Degeneration : **Weston Price**
This book is my absolute favourite dealing with nutrition, and although it does not have any instructions on what to eat, it is the research and the mind expanding findings on natural food versus processed food that make it worth reading.

Websites

www.beastskills.com : amazing site with tutorials on the basics and good articles, links, and other information.

www.tnation.com : Great website, more aimed at bodybuilding and general strength training than calisthenics, but has many excellent articles and is updated regularly.

www.gymnasticbodies.com : This site has lots of information and a very good forum, but is aimed primarily at the more serious strength training and bodyweight exercise practitioner.

www.rosstraining.com : Ross' site is great for motivational content and a no-nonsense approach to training. His writing style is very informative, and he has a great dislike for any fad equipment and for those people who are just out there to make a quick buck.

www.youtube.com : YouTube is home to so many videos and awesome physical displays that it is impossible to list all of them here. Simply do a search for calisthenics or bodyweight exercise and you will have lots of content to watch. It can be very good to learn from, or simply to get a little bit of motivation to inspire your own training.

www.marksdailyapple.com : Mark Sisson's site is one of the best for information about nutrition and the Paleolithic diet, which is one that I heavily subscribe to. A wealth of information here, and some very good links to other sites and books, products, etc.

www.myprotein.com : A very good website that I buy a number of things from, including liquid chalk, clothes, etc. Well worth a visit.

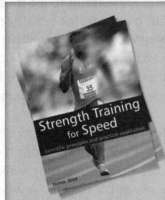
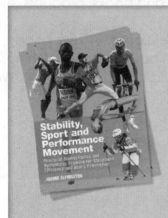
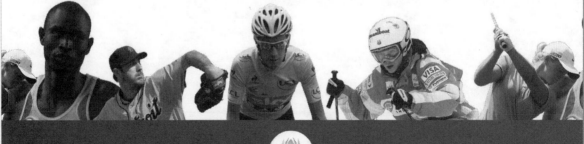